Psychoanalytic Perspec
Body Image, Shame, Ju
and Maternal Function

Have you ever been praised or criticized about your body or any part of it? With this question, participants of a research study were invited to share their experiences of body judgment. As participants described, the body is a carrier of messages and the source of judgmental experiences.

Psychoanalytic Perspectives on Gaze, Body Image, Shame, Judgment, and Maternal Function: Being and Belonging offers an insightful and engaging psychoanalytical account of experiences of shame and fear of rejection, explained through clinical vignettes and research participants' scripts. Exploring the findings from the individual and social standpoints, as well as the cultural and historical influences, Dr. Roth proposes that judgements are experienced as attacks, with the meaning attributed to the criticized body part, affecting the sense of self and forming a central point of the participants' identity trauma. Furthermore, that as guilt requires reparative action, shame requires an act of sacrifice to align the individual to the ideal and to preserve the matrix of belonging, thus explaining the participants' use of alienation as a defense.

This book will be of great interest to psychoanalysts and psychotherapists, as well as scholars of culture and religion. Giving a brief introduction to psychoanalytic concepts, with a full glossary, it will also appeal to the non-psychoanalytic reader interested in body image and how related perceptions and judgements can affect our own sense of Being and Belonging.

Lía A. Roth, PsyaD, was born in Argentina, where she studied psychology at the University of Buenos Aires. Once in the United States, she obtained a master's and a doctoral degree. In 2016, the International Psychoanalytic Association awarded Dr. Roth a Research Training Fellowship.

Psychoanalytic Perspectives on Gaze, Body Image, Shame, Judgment, and Maternal Function

Being and Belonging

Lía A. Roth

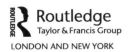

LONDON AND NEW YORK

First published 2020
by Routledge
2 Park Square, Milton Park, Abingdon, Oxon OX14 4RN

and by Routledge
52 Vanderbilt Avenue, New York, NY 10017

Routledge is an imprint of the Taylor & Francis Group, an informa business

British Library Cataloguing-in-Publication Data
A catalogue record for this book is available from the British Library

Library of Congress Cataloging-in-Publication Data
A catalog record for this book has been requested

ISBN: 978-0-367-46276-5 (hbk)
ISBN: 978-0-367-46275-8 (pbk)
ISBN: 978-1-003-02785-0 (ebk)

Typeset in Bembo
by Apex CoVantage, LLC

To my mother
Kaleka, sos mi luz

To my father
Gracias por darme una lengua
que maldice y bendice con precisión divina

To Harry
Darling, if I am always leaving you
it is because I am always returning to you

To Siggy
My teddy bear,
thank you for returning to my life in the shape of a dog

Have you ever been praised or criticized about your body?

Contents

Foreword

In 2008, I was diagnosed with skin cancer. One in every six women will have cancer in their lifetime. If I had to be one of them, I thought skin cancer was the easiest to tolerate. My tumor was a three-millimeter (mm) spot between my lip and my nose. After surgery I was left with a big Band-Aid covering the more than 40 stitches scar in the middle of my face. I did not want anyone to look at me. I could not stand their gaze. All I thought was people were looking my scar and not at me. I faded away behind a scar.

One day, someone told me that her aunt had had the same experience. As time went by, I learned about other people and acknowledged it was not just me making a big deal out of a little cancer spot. People were concerned about judgments received throughout their life regarding their hands, nose, breasts, teeth, or skin.

I realized the meaning of that Freudian statement about the body being the foundation of the self. I took a sabbatical year to mourn the person I was and to recreate myself. I went back to school to study how we make our own stories of identity in relation to body experiences. Since then, I have been collecting narratives of being praised or criticized for the way we look.

During a dinner party, I heard one of the first of these stories. A former professor from a local university 20 years my senior kept her hands out of my sight, under the table, covered by the napkin. I could not refrain from asking what was going on. I am not good at taming my curiosity. She told me that 40 years previously, she was teaching a little kid to read. This child told her she had the hands of a witch. Ever since, she had restrained from wearing rings and kept her hands out of sight. That instant, and by mere chance, I came up with the topic of my dissertation. We have all been there. But what do we do with those messages – how do we build our identity with or beyond them? The prompt came to me: Have you ever been praised or criticized about your body or any part of it? The answers the participants provided, together with clinical examples and personal experiences, powered this book into matters I was not aware I would end up visiting. It was most surprising to venture into such a commonplace topic and find it rich and extensive.

"No man ever steps in the same river twice"[1] (Borges, 1976). What I wrote for my dissertation is not exactly what I now present in the shape of a book.

It is a book that describes and explores the deep suffering of almost 20 participants and other individuals. Their stories and the other vignettes I present illuminate the discussion of how positive or negative judgments affect our sense of being and belonging. I have used different schools of thought for better exploration, always indicating from where I am coming.

When I was a child, most books and teachers would talk about "el hombre," the man indistinctly. At least I felt represented by that expression until someone had a different idea. I never questioned my sense of belonging until someone decided that "hombre" was not "ser humano;" *man* and *human being* were not the same thing. Gender difference came into the classrooms and turned simple conversations into an effort for those who would never want to hurt anyone's feelings. To show her inclusiveness, Argentinean President, Mrs. Kirchner, started her speeches by saying "a todos y todas,"[2] as if the word "all" would have never involved women and men alike. She called herself *presidenta* and most Argentinians went on to make a bigger effort into being politically correct. To every letter "o" – or neutrals "e, i, and u," – an "a" was appropriately added amending years of language oppression without consulting the Royal Spanish Dictionary (2020) where it clearly says that, for instance, the word "Presidenta" was incorporated in its Fifth edition of 1803.

How many times are we unaware of being oppressed until someone announces it? How many times do we feel oppressed when there is nothing but misinterpreted acts of kindness? We follow practices trying to amend an error that is a rhetoric of history and the remedy ends up being another manifestation of the disease. These are not innocent acts. Luckily, we have two ears. We can use one of those ears to listen to our heart, to respectfully recognize the difference, and to embrace it, which is the most challenging and honest act.

Then I moved to the United States and started to read in English. Reading was a mental struggle straining my eyes. I could not read a line just once and make sense of it. I had to go through the usage of *she/he* and *her/his*, like jumping hurdles on the way.

I know de Saussure said that language is an ongoing process. It seems years ago we were less sensitive, more tolerant. Sometimes I certainly believe it is more about being liable safe than a motion towards accommodating disparities. I'm not sure how all this helps science.

But these things, these attitudes and practices, tend to travel. Just last year, an Argentine soccer player was fined at an international match for using the N-word. *Negro, flaco, gordo* (negro, thin, fat) and others are terms of endearment in many Latin American countries. Indeed, words are not good or bad. What we decode from them may bring up feelings of mortification or praise. What we do with words is what could be injurious. Making differences breaks us apart. Many participants could not tell who said what. As Horton Cooley said, whether real or imaginary, judgments can bring feelings of mortification. It's not the words we use, it's what we do with them when we hear them and when we take part in spreading them. Words are just that – words.

This book does not pursue being politically correct. Nevertheless, I made an effort to comply with APA conventions, using *they* as singular. You will find the terms *they, them, their*, and *themself* instead of the previous *s/he* or *she or he* and similar constructions. This usage feels as close to a grammar offense as it can be. I hope readers do not feel they are jumping hurdles while reading this book.

I have called these sorties an attack on the link because, by dismembering the narrative in its parts and turning them into evil projections, the individual cannot move pass the disruption. There is no enriching interchange, no elaboration or work-through. The association between scholars is also disrupted as the lecturer loses agency. The attack takes the lecturer as prey, ceasing in their role. The lecturer becomes a freak who requires sacrificial cleansing. The listener is also in danger of abjection. Entering into contact or touching the abjected object could transfigure the innocent listener into an alienating "them" as well.

Abjection is what is purged when likeminded people bond following an idealized omniscient power, a mindset that creates strong boundaries, leaving out all that do not fit, all that is not suitable to their rhetoric. It is a disruption of the natural symbolic order. All those pieces left out, excluded, or repudiated are the abject – the superego's object of gratification.

In Chapter 5, I describe how at six years of age, I asked my mother about skin differences. I left this passage intact because my question was driven by the exemplary innocence of a child who has started to explore the world. I must have referred to the skin tone of my native nanny from Salta, north of Argentina, the orange shade of my father's Welsh skin, and the olive tint of my criolla mother, all the colors of people who were dear to me. In the Argentina of 1973, one did not come across Africans or Asians. The first time I saw an African American in Buenos Aires was in 1998. I approached him to say hi. We were at a restaurant. A toddler came running towards him, excited, and asked, "Who painted you?" With a smile he answered, "God did." Only days later, he ended up having an audience with the Argentine President, who wanted to learn more about his visit.

Furthermore, in Argentina of the 1970s, the level of poverty was not what it is now. The poor were respected as such and described as "Pobre pero honrado," which can be translated as "Poor but honorable." Thus, to those who read anything different in my use of the word *color* or any other term, I shall repeat: Words are not good or bad. What people make of them might be. When language is used in a perverse way, dialogue ends. Then, communication becomes dismembered into its emotional parts, which takes discourse adrift. Evil projections disrupt what otherwise could be an enriching encounter of minds. This dismembering can happen between a reader and their book. It can happen in interpersonal exchanges or among professionals. Let me whisper something to your ear: This book does not attempt to be right. I would rather have a dialogue.

Participants of this research also felt taken by a judgment that debased them. For the moment the judgment took place, they were no longer the teacher, the banker. They were the object of judgment, abjected by a superego that found them – in real or imaginary ways – unfit.

I grew up with a ladder positioned against the neighbor's fence as an escape route. How many times did we run away from home because my father had criticized the dictatorship? But we always returned home after each political storm. He was a best seller of political essays during the dictatorship years that ended in 1983. He was also appointed attorney general when he was in his thirties. We idealized the American idea of freedom. I believe that what kept us going was knowing that things were better, and freedom was possible somewhere "up north." As a foreign born, I have a different relationship with the American culture.

I mentioned how, through the years, I have listened to people's stories of body criticism. Friends from my country of origin could understand having a sensitive body part. They were astonished and could not accept that such body part would result in shame, avoidant behavior, or scapegoating among people residing in St. Louis, Missouri.

The idea for the chapter about the Puritans came to me when I was traveling. It is always refreshing to see something when we have taken a step back and found a new vantage point of view. I realized the deep suffering of the participants was not only about the judgments received. There is something in the individualism of the American culture, a society that originated from a separatist movement. Participants of my research resided in the Bible Belt where much of the history of North America took place, where American Indians sold their land and ended isolated into reservations. Africans were kept under chattel slavery; Dread Scott and others lost their legal battles for freedom;[3] and women continued the old practice of losing their maiden names to acquire their husband's, which symbolizes becoming their personal property, a system that has rejected anything that is different to the point of shunting some of its citizens. All those historical events gave shape and foundation to a worldview that is now the American culture.

There is a long practice of fundamentalism in those sections of the United States that make up the Bible Belt, an area in which, by history, Tanathos more than reason sets the absolute status of its citizens. Rooted in the separatist and Puritanism movement that did not include the Virgin Mary, American culture rejects difference. In that locus, participants felt there was something deeply sinister and wrong about them, something that debased them, something I called being a *freak*. For them, this meant being at risk of exclusion. They presented anxiety, isolation, alienation, avoidant behavior, and concealment. I have described the importance of shame, its differences from guilt, and how clever avoidant behavior and further defensive maneuvers safeguard both object and self.

The United States was not only colonized by the Puritans. The difference is that the Puritans arriving to the United States were usually healthier and more organized than their counterparts (Chaplin, 2001/2003). The first ones to arrive did not count on staying in America. I could imagine how they missed all the comforts of a village, compared to the open land they found in an uncolonized America. It was only successive generations that felt no melancholy over the Old Continent. The campaign to settle started with them (Chaplin, 2001/2003).

The hurtful acts associated with early American colonization are still embedded in the culture of the American society, where my study took place. Old acts are never forgotten. I believe they give shape – a special intensity to the shame presented by the participants.

The Puritan mindset is still active and widespread. Jung called scientism the control and manipulation of knowledge. When science is dogmatized and taken as Truth, then there is no advancement but repetition, no learning but indoctrination. Just a few days ago, I visited the president of a psychoanalytic institute. He expressed the need to follow dogma and tradition; I asked: Whatever happened to the Freudian values of wish and desire? He had no answer. It reminded me of how Freud used to say psychoanalysis is an art. There can be no art in the scientism of dogma and tradition.

Dogma and tradition create a protective space, where the most scared of individuals can live in peace. Everything is homogeneous, clean, known, and repetition of ritual takes place. It can have an atomistic effect. In the United States, there is an extreme form of American individualism. Unfortunately, this individualism comes at the price of a deficit in structural self – object relationship building that makes people vulnerable, particularly when they wish to belong.

I would like to thank the participants of my research study called Cracked Mirror, as well as the participants of this book, all of which will remain as anonymous contributors. Without your assistance, presence and patience I would have not made it.

I want to offer my deepest gratitude to Dr. Stephen Soldz and Dr. Marjorie Goodwin from Boston Graduate School of Psychoanalysis, as well as to Dr. Dirk Voss, professor of American History at the University of Missouri, for their assistance and availability. To María Maluf, María Ángeles Rivas, Mónica Blanco, Lucila Rosso, and my dear everlasting friend María Ladrón de Guevara. Diana Bellessi, thank you for believing in me and thank you for all the generous morning smiles from Picasso café employees where I wrote most of this book.

Lía A. Roth, St. Louis, MO

Notes

1 "Nadie baja dos veces a las aguas del mismo río" (Heraclito, Borges, 1976).
2 One should not confuse grammar with machismo. The use of masculine is general, and in no way refers to the masculine / feminine opposition. It is incorrect to make gender distinctions regardless of the number of individuals of each sex that are part of a group. In Spanish, the male gender is unmarked. Therefore, it can be used equally in reference

to being of female and male sexes. (Speech given by the former RAE's Director, Darío Villanueva, during the presentation of the book on Spanish style called, Libro de estilo de la lengua española: según la norma panhispánica, 2019). My translation.

3 Others, as Henrietta Wood sued Zebulon Ward for enslaving her after she earned her freedom. In April 17, 1878, the federal courtroom in Cincinnati, Ohio awarded her nearly $65,000 in present value (McDaniel, 2019).

1   Made out of crystal

"It's like I'm made out of crystal. People can look through me; and they all despise me," Mr. Whyte said. Mr. Whyte could not look me in the eyes. He kept holding his hat, as he wrinkled it between his hands while staring down to the floor. He was more than 40 years old when he started coming to sessions. Although tall, his somber walk with a bowed back made him appear rather small. His entire posture expressed the deep shame he was constantly feeling. He was terrorized by the belief that people tend to look at him, talking ill of him behind his back.

For years Mr. Whyte has been trying to avoid looking at his coworkers with the magical expectation that they, in turn, would not be able to see him. In the same manner, he isolated himself by using headphones. He believed his headphones stifled people's voices. My understanding was different. Those headphones were a counter-phobic object that mediated his relationship with the environment. The voices criticizing him were likely a projection of his own insufferable aggression he could not contain within. The headphones helped by stopping that projection.

He genuinely felt others could read his mind and had nothing good to say about him. It took him a while to understand it was his own aggression projected onto others that haunted him. Although the level of suffering may differ, Mr. Whyte's account is prototypical of many others. He wishes to belong, but his belief of self-inadequacy and weakness stops him short. He appears as symptomatic of an early fixation in the mirror stage of early development I will be exploring in this book.

This book is based on a qualitative research project I performed as part of my doctoral degree. I have also added vignettes from my clinical work and personal affairs. I believe the body is the vantage point of our existence, and the experience of belonging to a body is our sense of self. The body gives continuing support to our sense of self, starting every morning when we decide how to show ourselves to the world – our hair style, the way we dress, use make-up, inscribe tattoos, as much as the way we walk and make gestures. The rhythms we have are all an expression of how comfortable (or not) we feel with our bodies and the effect we want to make on others. One of the participants, Mrs. Byer, won a contest for the most beautiful eyes when she was five years old. She has been making her eyes up ever since. As a septuagenarian Jewish woman, she continues to find her beautiful blue eyes are a protective shield against criticism and discrimination.

Our body gives shape to our sense of self. Consequently, it also weighs in on the way we relate with one another. In Gogol's (1836/2014) *The Nose*, the Collegiate Assessor Kovalev wakes up one morning to realize his nose is gone. He eventually sees someone of much higher ranking than his getting into a fancy carriage. He realizes this decorated civil servant is his nose. Kovalev covers his face with a handkerchief after having lost the phallic symbol of his virtue. He feels dethroned by his own nose doing so much better than him.

Rostand's (1897/2009) *Cyrano de Bergerac*, that chivalrous, sharp musketeer that was as quick with his sword as he was with his mouth. Cyrano's nose was his scepter and orb . . .

> My nose is huge, enormous, vast!
> Listen, poor snub-nose, flathead,
> Empty headed meddler, know
> That I am proud possessing such appendice,
> 'This well known, a big nose is indicative
> Of a soul affable, and kind, and courteous,
> Liberal, brave, just like myself, and such
> As you can never dare to dream yourself,
> Because your foolish features are as bare
> Of pride, of passion, and of purity.
> (Rostand, Act 1, scene IV)

A nose can symbolize someone's best qualities, like in Bergerac's virtue, loyalty and bravery. It can also symbolize the biggest weakness and insecurities. Mr. Horowitz, one of the participants, felt his nose was so big people would not want to spend time with him. As with Cyrano de Bergerac, Mr. Horowitz did not feel a girl would be interested in him. In a Gogolian way, Mr. Horowitz's nose had a life of his own. He felt people were paying attention at his nose but could not see him as a person.

Mr. Horowitz is a successful businessman. He described himself as someone who used to be known for his nose. Currently, he would better describe himself as a "short, fat, bald guy." The nose "dominated my features for 20 years until it got fixed," shared Mr. Horowitz. He depicted his childhood nose as "Roman gothic, with a hook or a Jewish nose." He repeatedly broke his nose. Then, when he was around age 20, a doctor suggested surgery to allow proper breathing. Upon surgery, his nose reincarnated into "straight, normal. Perfect."

The nose is that protruding part at the center of the human face and takes about a third of its space. One can use it for guidance by following one's own nose, keep the nose clean, or win by a nose. One can turn their nose up at someone or be under someone's nose, stick their nose into something, or rub someone else's nose into something. For Bower (as cited in McNeil, 1998) the nose is always visible to assist in positioning objects or sensing whether it is they or we that are moving.

Noses provide human beings with the sense of smell, which is one of the earliest methods of perception. Infants can detect their mother's by scent soon after birth and adults identify their children or spouses by their aroma (Alperovitz, 2013). In an 1897 letter to William Fliess, Freud suggested "he turns up his nose = he regards himself as something particularly noble" (Masson, 1985, p. 279). Within East Asia, a big nose can be a sign of good fortune, or it has the negative connotation of showing the person is a foreigner. Pinocchio's nose would grow when he lied and was deceitful. His nose shows a negative attribute attached to big noses. In India's "earliest times, perhaps as far back as 3000 B.C., amputation of the nose was a traditional punishment for sexual misdemeanors" (Santoni-Rugiu & Sykes, 2007, p. 170).

Mr. Horowitz started the interview with laughter and asked for a repeat of the research probe. He needed time to master the interview situation. His laugh suggested feelings of inadequacy and hesitation about bringing memories of the past. "When I was a . . . When I was a kid, my nose got broke quite often for various reasons and I had a Roman gothic nose," he remembered. That Roman gothic nose was most painful for Mr. Horowitz. He shared this information on the second part of his statement. His emotional tone and memory brought up indicated the delicacy that was required from me to approach this topic:

> So, you get called names for it. Um. . . . It changes the way you'd look at yourself. It was enough where I didn't go . . . go dating anybody through high school. Didn't really think I should, 'cause I had this big nose. Got called everything from a Jewish nose, to a hooked nose, to a big nose. So you just use it as a joke instead of as a negative. So you'd make fun of your own . . . of my own, um . . . what I call . . . thought was a big nose.

When Cyrano de Bergerac falls in love with Roxane, his nose becomes the center of his doubts, as in the case of Mr. Horowitz. Their doubt is suggestive of an association between big noses and sexuality:

> This lengthy nose that goes wherever I will,
> Pokes yet a quarter mile ahead of me;
> Prevents me from being loved
> By even the poorest and most graceless of ladies.
> (Rostand, Act 1, scene V)

Mr. Horowitz's nose appears as a dominating feature. "So I took it away from the conversation. Since you go like old Jimmy Durante would say: 'That's no banana, that's my nose.' So if you came up with something funny or stupid, people would not be able to comment about it, since I did it first."

His use of humor as a defense mechanism implied the demands of his superego as representative of cultural values. His nose was not "normal." It was "disgusting," as Mr. Horowitz described it. It made him defective, unwanted. He felt identified with the socio-cultural qualities denoted by his big nose. Those qualities regulated his standing in the world and his social relations. If his nose was disgusting, he as person could not be any better. Mr. Horowitz avoided dating as a way of steering clear from repudiation.

Having broken his nose 25 times, a doctor suggested surgery: "I did not know it was important to me, but I probably wouldn't be where I'm at today. If it was still hooked, I might have stayed home and worked in a grocery store. I might have still been in (a small town). I probably would have been in out of the hole. . . . Probably I would have never dated girls."

Mr. Horowitz was in his early sixties at the time of the interview. The remainder of the participants of this research were individuals between 39 and 81 years old, all college-educated or above. The research started in April of 2016 with the prompt: "Have you ever been praised or criticized about your body or any part of it?" Our body and appearance have an impact on how we appraise ourselves and how we relate to our surroundings. How we feel about our body is influenced by the real or imagined judgments we receive throughout our lives, especially at times when we are particularly sensitive. It also has to do with the concepts of gaze, organic insufficiency, body image, and ultimately of our sense of being and belonging.

Participants talked about the size of their breast, height, old-looking hands, big noses, blue eyes, skin, clubfoot limp, gap between the front teeth, and their body shape. Everyone had a story to share. Their stories were an expression of a deep secret and secluded lifelong endurance. My research director, Dr. Stephen Soldz, and I were surprised to learn how profound and widespread this type of suffering is. Indeed, at one point or another in our lives, we've all been criticized about our body or a part of it. In addition, participants evinced having a particular body part prone to judgmental messages of a certain kind. Whether these messages are real or imagined makes no difference. Occasionally, judge and jury falls on the same person. As Mrs. Hughes acknowledged: "Sometimes we can be our worst enemies." In different instances, it can be someone else being critical. But the message – the judgment – must be timely and of significant value for impact.

For instance, since her twenties, Mrs. Teak has been convinced of having old-looking hands. She was a retired teacher at the time of the interview. As with a variety of professions, hers involved exposing her body in front of an audience. Mrs. Teak invested much of her time in the care of her hands. It was a way of dealing with her belief and doubts about the message and its meaning. For instance, she said, adults "are more critical of the way you look." Her friends would not be as honest because "they wouldn't want to hurt her feelings." Whereas "kids are brutally honest."

> Well, I've . . . Ah, I would say I've been criticized with my hands. I'm very, um . . . And it's been for a long time cause now that I am getting older. . . . But I still have very old hands for my age. . . . Um . . . When

I was a teacher, sometimes kids would comment, as I would write on the board, things like that. So . . . Um . . . I try to use . . . I think it . . . I think I . . . I became more self-conscious of it. . . . I've always kinda hurt my feelings and everything.

We start our lives by touching. Gradually, we learn there are things that can be touched and other ones that are untouchable. In India, Japan, and sundry parts of the world, the "untouchables" comprise the lowest social class. They attend occupations that make them unclean, impure, and outcasted (e.g., death-related jobs, cleaning of excrements, etc.).

Touch can happen skin to skin or it does not happen at all, as in the untouchables. In America, some withstand ostracism when they have done something considered out of mainstream. It is clearly observed when someone's nerve is touched while discussing politics. It happens when an employee loses face while walking away from their job with their box of personal belongings, never to return after being laid off. Being fired is more than just terminating an occupation. Losing the job means losing part of our identity, our social status, the associations established through employment. Many unemployed individuals find it difficult to resocialize past termination. They feel like they have lost their persona as a successful administrator, engineer, whatever. They do not know how to present themselves. Like one's name needs an occupation attached to it. Touch – and the untouchable – can be physical or symbolic.

Dr. Dillon was 50 years old when we met for the interview. He was tall, trim, and recently started to let his hair grow. There was an almost undetectable limp to his walk. His explanation for this was that one of his legs was shorter than the other one as well as the fact that he also had a clubfoot. But that was not the body part that concerned him:

I was with neighbor kids, cycling in the streets in Switzerland. And . . . Uh! It was a hot summer day so I took off my shirt and . . . and one of the kids turned around and said: "I would be ashamed if I had a fat belly like this one." And I was shocked! Truly shocked, I was not even aware that I had a belly.

Dr. Dillon, at the time a 14-year-old teenager, encountered an "athletic second-grade boy" that he barely knew. Receiving the message was like crashing against the western values embodied in the voice of a young boy that called him *fat*. Then Dr. Dillon said, "I think the kid was acting out something he heard and I think it has to do with the culture that you have to look fit." He felt he had no defense mechanism in place to respond. He had no way to say "Oh yeah! That's complete nonsense," as he did during the interview with me. Because the child spoke as he was turning his head to another youngster, it is also unclear whether the message was really directed at Dr. Dillon. Such a judgment "left a major impact on me. . . . I even remember that after almost 50 years. . . . I think that's sitting somewhere in the background of my head even if I'm consciously not aware of it."

The judgments that so deeply affected all participants, bringing feelings of shame, mostly emerged during puberty and adolescent years. For those that heard the judgment in later years, the problematic body part also surfaced in much later (e.g., psoriasis, wrinkles on neck, and dry skin). Their experience had an impressively deep and long-lasting repercussion. They all have been dealing with the sequelae ever since. Dr. Dillon admitted, "I even remembered it after almost 50 years. . . . It left a major impact on me." Dr. Kamala asserted, "The story is embedded over there and I, whenever I think of it, it's like a pinprick." Except for one, all stories were about negative judgments.

Where do we start?

In *On Narcissism*, Freud (1914/1953) refers to the infant as "His Majesty, the Baby," to express various issues. In the womb, a baby has warmth and security. All its needs are met and sustained in an oceanic[1] feeling of comfort. In this magic cosmic world, the unborn is at the center of their universe. It is crucial for the infant to continue to have a sense of fantasized omnipotence with the assistance of their first caregivers, as well as through an innate stimulus barrier that keeps them protected from the stimuli of the outside world.

Humans are born immature. All the perceptual senses (touch, sight, hearing, smell, taste) and social and cognitive skills need developing. Sight and gaze are not the same. Sartre (1943/1984) emphasizes how anything can bring the effect of a gaze. Gaze is preverbal, is drive ridden and related to partial objects whereas sight is developmentally later, related to our capacity to see and to somehow make sense or question what we are looking at following the reality principle – activity that is culturally affluent.

The establishment of perceptual neurosynapses starts at birth and develops gradually through different lines (Freud, 1965/2018) or networks (Biven, 1980), with successively increasing differentiation and in which "prior developmental structures are incorporated into later ones by hierarchic integration" (Inderbitzin & Levy, 2000, p. 218) in interaction with the environment.[2] These pathways, be it lines or networks, are susceptible to tensions of integration and fragmentation. Furthermore, this process is full of cultural and emotional influences. Children are born into a cultural world that preexists them. It is a world that influences them from before their birth takes place.

During the oral phase, a child gains a first edition of their body image.

> The oral body-ego exerts prehension and release (introjection and projection). From there evolves an oral ego organization in which attention and exploration of inner and outer space become the basis for the initial phase of object constancy. Only when self and object can be recognized as separated in space, can there be communication instead of communing.
>
> (Kestenberg, Marcus, Robbins, Berlowe, & Buelte, 1971, p. 750)

Mouths are the main source of our survival. We eat, communicate, feel, and learn using this part of the body. The initial contact with mother is made over mouth and nipples. While teeth stand for our sadistic and more cannibalistic impulses of introjection. One can be "armed to the teeth," "kick in the teeth," or react by "dropping one's teeth." Mr. Alem said having been criticized "several times over the course of the years" because of the gap between his teeth. In school, kids used to call him "snaggletooth." He recognizes he has his mother's teeth. His mother started wearing braces at age 60. Shortly after she did this, he started wondering about having braces as well. "It's a cosmetic thing."

Per Bowlby (1958), we come into the world with instinctual responses for attachment just as we have innate reflexes for physiological survival (e.g., grasping, patellar reflexes). Ultimately, these instinctual attachment responses foster our psychological development. These attachment responses include sucking, clinging, following, crying, and smiling. For instance, there are changes in pleasure, emotion, motivation, and satisfaction when a child drinks when thirsty. The feeling framework gives the experience its structure; and this happens in relation with a caregiver (Stern, as cited in Mellier, 2014). That feeling framework is the affective logic.

Each original encounter with an object is a diffuse experience of visual, tactile, acoustic, thermal, kinesthetic, cutaneous, and various sensory stimulations fused. The infant cannot access discrete objects yet. There is no differentiation between object, self, and context. Furthermore, in the cortex "the external body is represented *as an object*" among other external objects (Solms, 2013, p. 5). Only with maturity does the diffuse image differentiate into discrete objects and experiences, all of which are related to instinctual drives in the same fashion as the original undifferentiated image of the need–satisfying object.

Following Freud's pleasure[3] principle, an infant can feel a tension (e.g., the pain of hunger) building up. This tension requires an object for discharge satisfaction, action that eases the tension. When the object is present, a gratifying discharge takes place. If the object is not present, a detour happens. The delay that external reality imposes brings about two significant effects. One is the body being used for direct discharge, which is the archetype of all affective behavior. The second effect is a Freudian theoretical abstraction. The tension finds the memory trace of the needed object, and gratification takes place in a hallucinatory way. This hallucinatory image is the archetype of cognitive thought (Freud, 1925/1953; Rapaport, 1951/1996). Solms[4] (2013) considers the creation of representational "mental solids" are activated (or "cathected") by affective consciousness, enabling thought process.

The presence of maternal figure sustains cohesiveness, consistency, and helps regulate anxiety. Thus, the regression and use of hallucinatory sensory is also found in the transitional object. Be it a blanket, a thumb what acquires the maternal soothing qualities, or the introjection of such soothing power through a self-image.[5] Both these cases involve a gradual developmental strategy. It is a subterfuge that provides increased independence, allowing for a more stable sense of self when distant from mother. The separation–individuation process is progressive and everlasting. The creation of a system called individual cannot be considered in atomistic terms.

When a desire is realized, there is a discharge and a fulfillment. Affect is a quantity of energy susceptible to discharge, gratification, and displacement through desired conscious or unconscious specific actions. Each action provides a complementary qualitative tone. Affect and action are always working in conjunction. Whether the action is taken place as a motor discharge or innervation of a somatic body part, affect is a somatic sensation. That sensation can be pleasurable or not, conscious or unconscious, yet it always *affects* the ego.[6] Affect contains the mnemic traces of the somatic sensations experienced since birth, within a background provided by the caregiver. As such, it inscribes a pattern and is the earliest logic one can have. The background was there from even before the child was born. It is represented by parents that set up the crib, the colors of the room as they are expectant of delivery day. It is a cultural background full of wishes, fantasies, desires, and a measure of concerns.

Freud distinguished between identity of perception as earlier than identity of thought. From the economic point of view, identity of perception follows pleasure principle and seeks immediate discharge. It is free floating and does not require the mediation of the word. Within the primary process, affects do not require the use of signs for discharge (Chiozza, 1999). Conversely the secondary process is developmentally later, requires the use of word representations to achieve fulfillment by identity of thought. It is found in scientific and rational thinking (Akhtar, 2009). Reality principle governs the secondary process.

The affect is a plus, a force, a spare of any representation. It entails a qualitative aspect that adds meaning to every thought and action. The logic of affect never disappears. Rational thinking takes over with dominant power over emotions to secure safety and proper satisfaction by following the stricture of the reality principle. Adhering to the reality principle causes affective logic to banish. It is a matter of priorities and negotiations.

Affect can have a positive or a negative tone. What causes pleasure is welcomed, whereas things that are not pleasurable have a painful negative connotation. For instance, in Kleinian theory, an infant senses the discomfort of hunger as having a bad internal object, or a hate object. Hate is an affect originated by that force of discomfort that needs managing in order for the child to survive. Hate dawns from drives of self-preservation. It is discarded and handled by defense mechanisms. The self tends to push away what is threatening or not enjoyable. It can do this by using different defenses, like splitting. Splitting, denial, and reversal into its opposite are primitive ways of handling aggression.

For Ana Freud, projection and introjection come later in the development. Sigmund Freud depicted projection as the defensive mechanism that explained paranoia (Freud, 1896/1953). On the contrary, Melanie Klein (1929/1990) considered it a mechanism common in play of normal infancy. While Freud considered the infant as being in pure pleasurable state, Klein thought the infant contained good and bad objects.

The development of the infant is governed by the mechanisms of introjection and projection. For Klein from the beginning, the ego introjects 'good' and 'bad' objects, for both of which its mother's breast is the prototype. A child that can easily obtain pleasure from a breast, will find that breast to be a good object. A breast that requires a greater effort to make it work is a bad object. It is frustrating to deal with it. It is not only frustration that makes an object good or bad. The baby projects its own aggression on to these objects charging them with affect, turning them "bad." The child conceives them as being dangerous persecutors and fears they could be devoured by them.

> Scoop out the inside of its body, cut it to pieces, poison it – in short, compassing its destruction by all the means which sadism can devise. These imagos, which are a phantastically distorted picture of the real objects upon which they are based, are installed by it not only in the outside world but, by the process of incorporation, also within the ego.
>
> (Klein, 1935/1990, p. 145)

In 1987, Sandler conceptualized projection as the mechanism by which an unbearable unconscious instance (affect, idea, or drive aim) becomes a conscious object representation, thus, perceived as coming from outside the self. Projection, projective identification, splitting, regression, denial, and somatization are all defense mechanisms mobilized by forfeit of loss of harmony or threats to self-constancy, whether the threat is internal or not.

In different occasions, Freud depicted the representative agency of the drive as formed by two elements: (1) a representation or idea, and (2) a quantitative factor. This quantitative factor is the drive's energy, a "quota of affect" (Chiozza, 1999). A word-representation can be broken apart from its qualitative quantum, leaving the representation as innocent as Freud described in *Little Hans* (1909/1953). By the mechanism of displacement and condensation – which are two Freudian mechanisms comparable to Lacan's discourse metaphor and metonymy – the qualitative quantum can attach itself to another object representation or memory trace.[7] Little Hans (Freud, 1909/1953) displaced the aggression towards his father onto an animal, forming a false link. Through this tactic, Little Hans was afraid of horses, and could still maintain a warm relationship with his father.

Condensation and displacement are two basic modes of affect transformation of the unconscious processes, thus, not limited to phobia. Freud (1900/1953) first described condensation in *The Interpretation of Dreams* as a way of surpassing the dream censorship. It is a synecdoche, a nodal point of affective energies and imagery that can have more than one association when analyzed. Jokes, faux pas, and additional symptoms can all be a result of condensation and displacement. In Lacanian terms, condensation is assimilated to metaphor and displacement to metonymy emphasizing the analogy between, the mechanisms of the unconscious and those of language (Laplanche & Pontalis, 2018). Therefore, what Freud called displacement and Lacan named metonymy is the diachronic – horizontal – association of signs that happens in observable terms. For instance, it can be the combination of words used one after the other. On the contrary, metaphor refers to de Saussure's – vertical relationship. It is a relationship that happens in absentia, and coincides with what Freud called "condensation." In a joke or faux pas, a person says one thing (metonymy) but means another (metaphor).

Freud utilized the word *Trieb* to refer to what we now call "drive" (de Mijolla-Mellor, 2005). In German, *Trieb* means instinct, fuel, motor force or driving force. Freud drew on Schilder's (Freud & Jung, 1974/1994) poem "Die Welt-weisen" ("The Philosophers"):

> Quite temporarily
> While waiting for philosophy
> To take the world in hand,
> Hunger and love command.

As Schilder did, Freud recognized love and hunger as the two most powerful forces. Thus, we regularly use *love* to refer to the sexual drives and *hunger* as representative of the drives for self-preservation, also called "aggressive drive."

At the beginning, there is a dyad.[8] There is no boundary between me and not me. From the start, the ego is autoerotic. A person can find satisfaction in their own body or a part of it. Love is originally narcissistic and associated with sexual forces or drives. It chooses objects that can satisfy the drive – objects that can be incorporated. Object choice can be anaclitic or narcissistic. Mother is the first anaclitic choice and considered prototype of subsequent object-choices. Freud (1914/1953) tallied narcissistic love choices as: The person I once was, the person I want to be, the person I am, or someone that is a part of myself. Mother is the first object of love. Love objects, because they are narcissistic, make us feel better – even whole. Adults call it romantic passion.

Lacan (1958) noticed desire is what remains after need is subtracted from demand (Demand-need=desire). In the example of feeding the child, the object of satisfaction is the breastfeeding. Yet, in offering a breast, a parent also offers care, warmth, and the fact that they are cathecting, thinking, and caring for their child. Thus, every demand is ultimately a demand for love. While drive can find its satisfaction in an object (Freud), or through the path towards the object (Lacan), desire is a force, a movement, a field, never quite satisfied. The pleasure principle inhibits the search for pleasure beyond certain levels. Jouissance comes to dethrone the limits of pleasure principle. Desire is a defense against the jouissance. In jouissance, there is a pleasure beyond pleasure principle. Lacan (2009a) called *jouissance* the pleasure in suffering and symptoms, while Freud named it as the primary gain in illness, although these two things are not necessarily the same (Evans, 1996). In desire, there is always a search for something else. Once gratification takes place, the search for satisfaction continues, be it creatively or by repetition.

Mrs. Hoocker was more than 65 years old, 67 inches tall, and 109 pounds. She stated never having been as thin as she was at the time of our interview. One of the first things that surprised me from Mrs. Hoocker's narrative was her quick, playful, and vibrant use of language. Gestures, onomatopoeia, and speech were simultaneously concocted together for maximum expression. Keeping up with her speed proved a laborious listening practice.

The first time I asked Mrs. Hoocker if she had ever been criticized or praised for the way she looks, she pulled her shirt open and showed me her breasts. "Now that I've lost weight, they are flat." In doing so, she was making me feel the horror of castration: The breasts that were no longer there. Simultaneously, Mrs. Hoocker was foreclosing or denying her own experience of such feelings. Much of Mrs. Hoocker's identity narrative has to do with developing early and carrying DDD-size breasts. "I was tall. So, hormonal meant that I matured very fast, so I developed all my feminine organs very fast, so that included my bust."

Female breasts are culturally sexualized. In Western cultures, women with big breasts are considered sexy, or even prostitutes with poor intellectual connotations. They are celebrated as much as condemned. At the beginning of the interview, Mrs. Hoocker alluded to her breasts in proper, educated words. She started by calling them her "bust," though in due course, she referred to them as breasts, boobs, or titties. Each term enclosed the distinctive intensity of a memory. Her own girlfriends from school called her "Big Boobies Hoocker;" whereas men used terms with a more "sexual" connotation, evoking her fear of being perceived as a prostitute as her own last name would imply. There are good breasts, bad breasts (Klein, 1931/1990), and wrong breasts (Sullivan, 1953).

For Mrs. Hoocker, breasts appear as a prime point of contact with her social surrounding. She can say now that she felt bullied as a child. Back then, she did not have a word to name how she felt. She just knew she was avoiding people who might set off her alarms calling them "Dirty Old Men." She dreaded going into elevators by herself as she presumed men would try to touch her with their elbows, blaming it on the compact space between them. Her breasts were also a gateway, as she learned to classify those who were safe to be with from those who made her feel threatened, depending on age and behavior. She married the only one that did not make comments about her breasts. This strategy allowed her to anticipate and shelter herself in order to circumvent potential conflicts and feelings of disgust.

Mrs. Hoocker used a variety of defense mechanisms, from denial to omnipotent control and isolation. At times, she tried not to pay too much attention. She concealed parts of her body and herself whenever possible. She hid her ample bosom between her arms and often checked her cleavage, observing herself in a narcissistic way. In doing so, she was both the exhibitionist and the voyeur. In her thirties, she underwent breast reduction surgery.

It wasn't easy, but humor provided a positive protective layer at the moment of facing the most dramatic and hurtful memories. Occasionally, I felt that the descriptions made by Mrs. Hoocker during the interview had an educational resemblance. She bragged about her ability to hold a six-pack with her bosom. Clearly, as I learned during the interview, I am scarcely endowed and therefore unprepared to have the slightest idea to understand what that means.

Horton Cooley (1902/1922) suggested self-awareness is an emotional effect product of real or imagined judgments that we receive from others. Mrs. Hoocker had to handle her own body parameters, the perception of how others reacted in real or imaginary ways to her body, as well as the resulting value meaning of social judgments for her own sense of identity. Social judgments that came in an imaginary way suggest they are the result of projective identification. Mrs. Hoocker stated that she married the only man who never looked at her breasts or made any mention of them.

For Skeat (1910, p. 342), to love means to covet. Love is an early unquestionable possession supported on the biological truth of uterine life. The mother-infant dyad changes from a mother who first possesses her child to one who yearns for them and vice versa for the infant. From this primary attachment comes our sense of belonging. Eventually, to love will mean to yearn for and to have one another. In adulthood, love is an object of choice that involves mutual trust and confidence that the bond is strong enough to secure each other's well-being. This adult form of love is the closest aspiration in later life to that early oceanic feeling we once experienced in the womb.

Since Freud's (1915/1953) *Papers on Metapsychology*, psychoanalysis has gone beyond simply describing behavior. Analytical abstractions are understood to better explain mental processes. One such abstraction is Freudian drive theory; another one is Kleinian object relations theory. Following Klein (1931/1990), in psychoanalysis, we use the term *object* to indicate a person or thing, whether real or imagined, that is of interest for the satisfaction of a drive. There are a diverse of ways to use the term object (e.g., good-bad object, partial-full object, etc.). Object relations are present from birth.

Freudian theory conceptualizes the ego and superego as developing with maturity and exposure to reality, whereas for Melanie Klein (1931/1990), there is a primitive ego and superego from birth. Both Lacan and Klein conceptualized the ego as containment of identifications. A containment keeps an inscription of all the early experiences of handling received. Identification is to unconsciously take in, introjecting, qualities of another person. For instance, a daughter smiling like her father or a victim behaving as the aggressive perpetrator would. Of course, Klein was concerned with internal objects and intrapsychic processes. Lacan, with the relation of the imaginary, the symbolic, and the real, did not limit himself to what is internal. Freud, rather, conceptualized the ego as the reservoir of the drives and defense mechanisms, as well as a representative of reality. Henceforward, he changed and realized the id was the reservoir of the drives.

From birth, there is an unconscious phantasy of omnipotence. A baby believes that whether internal or not, they have total power over the universe (Freud, 1908/1953). Whereas for Klein (1921/1990) the pain of hunger is felt in the body (in the ego) as a bad internal object. An effective caregiver will relieve the pain by providing appropriate actions. These actions happen within that special dyadic relationship a caregiver and her baby have, in which the symbiotic relationship makes them as one.

The caregiver interprets her baby's condition to generate whichever action is deemed appropriate. Every touch, every pain or pleasure felt in the skin is associated with the mother's correlative capacity for emotional containment and transformation into actions. Mother is the person in the role of caregiver. In my clinical work with Hispanic immigrants, patients have emphasized the importance of the biological mother in spite of their unavailability to deliver care. I am, thus, using the words caregiver and mother interchangeably.

Dr. Kamala was an international student when I interviewed her for the research. Somber years followed when, as a child, she lost her mother to a schizophrenic outbreak. She was either distant, "quiet and reserved," or "throwing temper tantrums." She hid from the frustrating reality into the safety of her imagination, and her studies:

> So, I concentrated on doing more and more, putting in more and more effort in my studies so that I get some recognition somewhere, and if – if there's no peace at home, at least in school, I'm happy and, uh, people recognize my talent.

It appears that Dr. Kamala realized the drawbacks of being short in temporal association with her mother's schizophrenic outbreak. Her hard work to be recognized, to be accepted could also be a way of searching for her mother's gaze:

> My mother was a very good student. She always topped not only in school, but also in the state and the country level so, um, she was always well recognized, and everybody praised her.

Mothering is a role and a responsibility. For the infant, mother is a cathectic investment. At first, mother is not just an external object, an image or a representation but – in the bests of cases – an emotional experience of being soothed, cared and provided. It is an experience eventually organized under the representation of a mother. But newborns relate to part objects. They relate to the breast, to a piece of mother's clothing, . . . not to the full person.

When the newborn begins to perceive its mother, it is unable to distinguish temporary absence from enduring loss; thus, from the moment the mother is out of sight, the baby behaves as if it is never going to see her again. Repeated experiences of satisfaction have created this object, the mother, which, as need arises, is intensely cathected in a way that might be described as nostalgic. From this moment on, in Freud's view, object-loss provokes psychic pain, while anxiety is the reaction to the danger associated with that loss. At this stage, the newborn experiences fragmentation anxiety. Sadness arises whenever reality-testing forces, an acknowledgment that the object has been lost. In its various forms, object-loss becomes the prototype of later anxieties (de Mijolla-Mellor, 2005, p. 99).

For Klein (1931/1990), the illusion of safety, control, and integration is achieved through the good breast provided by the mother. What the baby perceives is the discomfort vanishing, for instance, with a breast that is good because it has the capacity to ease the pain. As the infant matures, it gives way to the constrictions of reality. The infant accepts the distance from the mother by crafting an object to maintain the idea of mother's presence when she is out of sight. At the same time, transitional object is the expression of the child's egocentrism. This artifice sustains the child's feeling of constancy and continuity. A child is vulnerable without this strategy. Vulnerable, their sense of being alive and capable of self-soothing is at stake. Erikson (1980) called his first developmental stage trust vs. mistrust. Thenceforward, this translates in self doubt about their capacity to manage their anxiety, and to do and be well.

Mother is the primordial object. After the oceanic experience of intrauterine life, the dyadic relationship forms the basis of the most primitive source of cohesiveness an individual can have. Thus, the soothing effect and the yearn to reencounter the affair once had with mother. The child does not yearn for the mother per se, but for the experience of well-being found in the maternal relationship. The omnipotence and magical thinking of the affective logic turns the dyadic relationship into the closest creation to the oceanic feeling once felt. It is at the core of our narcissism, although taking different forms in accordance to the developmental stage and needs.

An imago is more than an image or a representation. It is an idealized creation made in early childhood that remains somehow unaltered throughout life. It is a narcissistic maneuver. Thus, the longing for the experience once felt within the dyadic space takes many forms. Blanket, thumb, self-image, sense of belonging are all narcissistic sources of cohesiveness or good gestalt. These are all, in different developmental proportion, soothing transitional objects anaclitically constructed.

Effective early care provides strength and continuity to the primitive ego. Such capacity allows the creation of representations for the self. Little frustrations that happen here and there can be tolerated by having that strength that first spurs from the dyadic relationship, and then slowly gains independency from it by using transitional objects, gaining object constancy or by the creation of a self-representation at the mirror stage as it happens later. Marking the creation of an independent system. However, being is belonging.

I have mentioned how mother at times is not available and her absence leaves the infant in jeopardy. There are also phantasies of engulfment at staying within the dyad. Thus, the child's need for separation, differentiation, and independence is not only by the father's precepts of the Oedipus Complex. Identification and transitional objects allow the child to move away from the dyad, avoiding the phantasies of engulfment without giving away the sense of security and wholeness once felt.

The small frustrations are an opportunity for the child to adapt. By confronting the limits of reality, a child gains ego resources. From this motive springs the importance of playing with toys to achieve classification, reversibility, and seriation within temporal-spatial dimensions. Unfortunately, through computers, tablets, smartphones, and other technological devices, children under five years of age are growing up without achieving their full potential. In the United States 81% of the population has a smartphone, and younger people are more likely to use technology (Silver, 2019). Children exposed to technology at an early age present loneliness and isolation, disorders of vision, reduced attention span and reduced sleeping time, increased sedentarism and obesity, and increased aggression (Bavelier, Green, & Dye, 2010; Chen et al., 2019). It affects the development of ego resources used, for instance, to regulate anxiety; as well as the development of motor, cognitive, and social skills. The World Health Organization (2019) is requesting parents to reduce children exposure to technological devices to one hour a day.

Mrs. Clayton recently started therapy. She was terrorized about being left by her partner. She had an abusive rearing. Mrs. Clayton's description of her father was a list of suitable bad words. In the same way, she had nothing positive to say about her mother. Spotnitz (1961) narcissistic defense suggests that after an early injury, the first objects are protected by love to avoid hurting them. Destroying these first objects would be threatening to the infant. Mrs. Clayton presented a long feeling of frustration, aggression, self-loathing, and loss of hope of anything better coming her way. She questioned whether she deserved her partner's love and often did everything at hand to sabotage that relationship. Her behavior with her current partner is a theater for the past phantoms of primary relationships to display through repetition; the actualization of that love-hate ambivalence now in association with what her partner brings to the table; the actual healthy relationship that is taking place whenever they both find health moments; as well as the expectancies and dreads that come once contemplating their future together.

When I interviewed Mr. Galeno, he had lived with psoriasis for 20 years. His psoriasis had spread all over his body, except for part of his face and his genitalia. He stated he first contracted psoriasis after his fiancé passed away in a traffic accident. It was as if his fiancé had been a skin layer he lost when she passed away. For Bick and Harris (1968/2011), the skin gathers the undifferentiated body parts in a desperate defense of integration and in order to avoid falling apart or being torn away. Skin can express someone's suffering even before the development of verbal language (Ungar, 2012).

Skin is considered a person's self-other boundary. It also has seven additional functions rendered by Anzieu-Premmereur (2015) as maintenance, containment, protection, individuation, intersensoriality, sexualization, libidinal recharging, and inscription. For Anzieu (2007), the body ego is first a skin ego. Porter, Beuf, Lerner, and Nordlund (1986) found that individuals with psoriasis present lower self-esteem and more prejudice due to the visibility of their skin condition.

"When I'm going out with somebody and I get past that, there's always the remark of: 'You know, you're really good-looking,' once I get pass the psoriasis. . . . So it's kind of a Catch-22 in the sense that you're getting a compliment, but it's not. It's kind of a backward compliment in a lot of ways." A compliment is a Catch-22. Mr. Galeno can recognize a negative element hidden beneath a flattering remark. He explained this Catch-22 while holding his right hand in a half fist. Compliments are a slap in the face. His face is one of the very few places where he is almost free of psoriasis.

Mr. Galeno makes an effort to control how people may look at him:

> I spend a lot of time primping and prepping myself so I look as good as I can. You know, skin-wise and stuff like that. So, uh, . . . every morning, um . . . I have to be careful with showers. If I take a 10-minute shower, then I look horrible and I feel horrible. It's a nightmare! Psoriasis and water don't mix very well. So, if I take it, if I do bathe, and when I do bathe . . . it just takes me an hour each time. Then I gotta make sure (that) my nails don't get fungus . . .

When asked about his earliest memory, Mr. Galeno said: "I remember, uh . . . my brother being in a crib and me, being on a mattress." In Mr. Galeno's memory, his brother had a holding environment whereas he was just on a mattress. The loneliness of an open space called mattress, left neglected where there was and still is no one to hold him. His memory expressed the absence of a supporting environment. With the psoriasis, he feels nobody dares touch him.

The infant considers discomfort as coming from malicious bad objects. For Melanie Klein (1931/1990) infants are swamped by a world of good and bad object relations causing bodily sensations that require attention. Through all the bodily maneuvers performed to alleviate the discomfort, the infant experiences, learns, adapts, and accumulates sense data, developing perceptual senses and cognitive-motor skills. Alongside every satisfactory motor action, there is a pleasant feeling. It is a feeling that pushes to repeat the action (Piaget, 1979). The operation is repeated no longer just for the sake of survival but for jubilation. A mother's breast is no longer used solely for nourishment but for the pleasant feeling gained around the mouth. Freud recognized this as the sexual drives being anaclitically leaning on the drives of self-preservation. As anaclitic, it is supported or attached to someone or something. Sexual drives find support in the drives of self-preservation to find their object and satisfaction. During breastfeeding, the first experience satisfies the hunger (self-preservation). Thereafter, it satisfies the sexual demand of the erogenous zone the mouth is. The first fulfillment inscribes a level of satisfaction that can never be replicated again. Nevertheless, people don't give up the search for pleasure easily.

Freud defined the drive as an internal constant force or pressure that has a source, an aim, and an object. This pressure appears in the mind as a demand for work, to bring satisfaction, and ease the discomfort. The drive stands in the limit between the body and the mind. It is "the concept on the frontier between the somatic and the mental . . ., the psychical representative of organic forces" (Freud, 1915/1953, p. 2455). The source of the drive is the part of the body where the somatic process occurs. The aim is to fulfill the demand and cease the discomfort. The object is the most variable element (e.g., a part of the body, an external object, a fantasy . . .). The object can be real or imagined, as when we daydream. At first, the object is represented as a thing representation, following identity of perception of the primary process. Once the child enters into language, the object achieves word-representation following identity of thought.

In every satisfaction, there is an array of affect, somatic, and representational processes working. In the example of the infant and the mother's breast, the source was the mouth, making it an oral drive that ceases with the satisfaction found through the breast or something used in its place, such as the thumb. The soothing maternal qualities are transmuted and internalized as a regulatory trick to preserve some of her qualities – and the service they provide – even when she is not present. The creation of a transitional object is a tactic that involves a hallucinatory regressive satisfaction as discussed above.

I have been referring to the drives as classified as sexual or for self-preservation. In "Beyond the Pleasure Principle" (Freud, 1920/1953), the antithesis continued as death and love drives, also known as Thanatos and Eros. Sexual drives are drives for self-preservation that deviated in their aim. Through the drives for self-preservation, sexual drives find their source, aim, and object. Self-preservation drives admit the acceptance of reality principle because only real objects can ensure our survival. On the contrary, sexual drives are free to follow the pleasure principle in its continuum of pleasure-displeasure. Breastfeeding is a biological need, but the act of sucking the breast gives pleasure to the mouth, turning it into an erogenous zone. For Lacan, beyond the pleasure principle a quantum of the jouissance can surprise us, field in which desire acts as a defense mechanism.

Eventually, the object used for satisfaction (e.g., breast) can be replaced. For instance, by using the thumb for discharge, gratification, and to represent the cohesive sense provided by the mother readily available. Sexual drives originate from numerous pleasure-sensitive body parts that become erogenous zones. They begin by working independently from one another to achieve organ pleasure. Eventually, they assist preparing body and mind for the primacy of genital satisfaction. Sexual drives continue to compel to seek satisfaction throughout our lives.

The drives can easily be in conflict with one another. Therefore, defense mechanisms come to assist the ego in managing manifold realities and myriad conflicts. Adequate actions for satisfaction progressively develop by exposure to incremental needs of adaptation. Defense mechanisms also go evolving. With time, anxiety acquires a degree of textures and tones. Fixation points and their correspondent defense mechanisms mark developmental stages and define psychical structure. Some people make more use of some type of defenses; others use different ones.

Freud (1915/1953) indicates the earliest defenses are splitting and reversal into its opposites (e.g., active-passive, sadism-masochism, exhibitionist-voyeur). These pairs of opposites foresee the possibility of the drive turning upon the subject's own self. Another early defense mechanism worthy of mentioning is repression. The next chapter on gaze makes use of these defense mechanisms and others.

Notes

1 The oceanic feeling is an experience of limitlessness and an all-embracing bond with the universe. Freud borrowed the term *oceanic* from Romain Rolland. "It consists of peculiar feeling, which he himself is never without . . . a sensation of 'eternity,' a feeling as of something limitless, unbounded – as it were, *oceanic*" (Freud, 1930/1953, p. 64)

2 The idea of biological integration through maturity and in interaction with the cultural world started over a century ago and remains valid. The corpus of psychoanalytic theory has a variety of conceptualizations on the topic. Nevertheless, the body, its structures, and drives (for ego or object relations) as well as the capacity for internalization are all part of developmental process in one way or another.

3 In psychoanalysis there are many colloquial words that have a specific conceptual meaning. The early infantile pleasure does not convey the absence of pain, nor does the pleasure principle mean to focus on pleasure seeking. In Instincts and their vicissitudes (1905) Freud says "I must insist that a feeling of tension necessarily involves unpleasure." In other words, the libido – that force that pushes the drive to seek gratification – has an unpleasant charge. The seeking force is towards discharge and gratification. Furthermore, it is within the pleasure principle that repetition and jouissance take place; and what is pleasure for one system can be unpleasurable for the other.

4 For Solms (2013), the ego is an unconscious instance, whereas Freud considered it to be conscious.

5 I will explain this further in the last chapter as it involves comparing different schools of thought.

6 "Freud seems not to distinguish between the terms affect, emotion, and feeling" Chiozza, 1999, p. 111). Etymologically, the term affect means "to influence, or act upon someone or to affect" (Blánquez Fraile as cited by Chiozza, 1999, p. 111). Thus, an affect is something that affects the ego. Whereas the word emotion refers to something that is moving (in Spanish, conmover), "to cause emotion." Feeling means "sensation," "to perceive through the senses," and "to realize," "to think, to give an opinion" (Blánquez Fraile as cited by Chiozza, 1999, p. 111).

7 Lacan's review of Freudian works comprises three registers. Thus, several of his terms are comparable but not equal. Freud's theory is a drive theory, whereas Lacan considered desire (also translated as wish) as the constant force.

8 There are different theories regarding when and how the infant access discrete objects. Thus, whether the relation with the caregiver is dyadic, symbiotic or merging.

2 The body image

During early infancy, there is no dichotomy of body and mind, but a single, undifferentiated experience of sucking-sensing-feeling-phantasying (Isaacs, 1948, p. 86; Ogden, 2011, p. 934). Freud characterized this period as being under the supremacy of the primary process. In the primary process, there is no discrimination of the external world, no sense of time, of contradiction or negation, and impulses are not coordinated. In the primary process the drive runs as free energy towards immediate gratification and discharge.

Freud (1923/1953) described the importance of the body as a cornerstone of ego development. The body is a foundational fact. Kristeva (1985) described the infant as semiotic. Preverbal language makes use of sensations, postures, rhythms, gestures, and visceral processes for a mother to interpret, give meaning to, and take action. Infants are rocked, washed, and handled in various ways. Each touch, every pain or pleasure felt in the skin is associated with the mother's correlative capacity for emotional containment and transformation into appropriate actions. In doing so, each feeling state is transmuted into states of mind. Different states of the baby are translated into emotions, unconscious wishes or beliefs (e.g., phantasies) a mother's child creates for themselves and will keep for most of their life. The capacity to use the memory traces of these early experiences is the essence of thinking. To think is to elaborate through symbolization. New memories can be added, broadening the self states, but the first memories – whether positive or negative – usually have an indelible strength.

Early memories, as Mr. Galeno showed, can offer a sort of theater for the self, between the subject and its object of desire. This theater stands as the psychic reality of our universe. It can be unconscious and hallucinatory as when we are dreaming. It can also be a daydream, and part of the preconscious-conscious system. In both cases, a drive finds its satisfaction, whether it is aggressive, erotic, or an expression of narcissistic grandeur.

Following Abraham (1966), Freud envisioned child development as going through stages (oral, anal, genital, and phallic). Every way of satisfaction, object relation, activity/passivity, perception, learning, and so on is consequential to a certain level of psychological organizational stage. It is interesting to notice that although psychologists understand the primacy of the mirror stage in the formation of the ego, the mirror stage has never been regularly included among the stages of maturity. In the same manner, it has not been regularly considered a fixation point, regardless of the level of suffering found in clinical work, such as with Mr. Whyte and many of the participants of this study.

Each developmental stage claims an erogenous zone as its primary organizer. Drive organization depends on the tribulation and success of the maturational processes. A fixation point is a position along the maturity process in which a partial drive leaves a mark. An overflow of energy the child cannot processed creates the fixation point. A fixation point can also be created due to certain unwillingness to give up a way of satisfaction. Under stress, we may return to this point. When confronted with extreme levels of affect, the inability to properly handle that economic charge may result in a regression. Returning to a previous psychosomatic functioning organization awakens the qualities of the self, its ways of satisfaction, and relating, as well as a set of defense mechanisms, concomitant effects, and phantasies proper of that stage the individual returns to. Mr. Whyte felt he was made out of crystal. That appears as an early developmental failure that had reverberations in his ability to find a positive image in the looking glass or when mirroring against other people. Freud would say that the persecutory experience has a narcissistic source. In terms of Melanie Klein, the projected bad parts of the self turn persecutory.

Mother is the very first mirror a baby has. Some people can look at themselves in the mirror experiencing estrangement for hours. As if their mirror had been cracked, they seem unable to find a healthy image for themselves, and the images received from others are full of disapproving messages. In the case of Mr. Whyte, he had reached a fixation point that was organized based on the gaze as the primary organizer erogenous zone. His own projections were damaging and paranoid. For Sartre (1943/1984), being watched makes us self-conscious. For Lacan, gaze is a distortion of vision. Vision is to look and to be looked at. The latter is paralyzing because it involves the big Other. In the field of vision, gaze is also conceptualized as the *object petit a* by the imaginary desire of the pre-linguistic other. It is the jouissance, as the superego has not been yet internalized. Gaze experience can happen through a variety of perceptual senses, like when Mr. Whyte heard others speaking ill about him behind his back, or felt others condemning him with their eyes. Gaze leaves a feeling of desecration indicating the action of the sadistic superego falling over us. But gaze is developmentally earlier than the superego proper.

I have been explaining the importance of appropriate maternal care. When starting to come out from the close dependent relation with their mother, the child begins discovering their own body. Global and spatial neuropathways carry data to the brain for processing (Liu, Yuan, Ding, Xu, & Long, 2017). The coordination of touch and sight allows a child to check form, size, weight, and surface qualities of an object as abstract visual information. Hands, ears, and eyes are usually in sync, or it results in clumsy movements. To overcome clumsiness, the child creates a visual map of their self in an environment, a primitive body schema (*Körperschema*, Schilder, 1935). Like a map, the outline of the body allows turning of the head so that visual information does not disturb movement when reaching toward something (Hyvärinen, Walthes, Jacob,

Chaplin, & Leonhardt, 2014). "Gradually, the earlier unmentalized cathexis of mouth, hands, and eyes get integrated into a primitive 'body schema' that, in turn, is underscored by perceptually locating the musculoskeletal pleasure of crawling and upright locomotion" (Akhtar, 2009, p. 39).

As with any behavior, visual motor activities involve an emotional tone, which is ongoing and adaptive. An emotional flow can start as much as interrupt an activity. In the case of Mr. Whyte, he wore headphones and eyeglasses to control his relationship with his work environment and his self-feeling. Only then was he able to do his job. He felt more comfortable with his younger children, believing he had lost the respect of his adolescent child.

As a baby is held by its mother, they can feel and see her attentive presence. Her face is the baby's first face. A mother looks at her baby and her look is not mere sight. It is a driven gaze. That gaze cathects the baby's body. She looks at her baby as her phallic object, which supports the child's sense of early grandiosity. A mother felt to be absent by her child leaves an indelible mark that announces the formation of a vulnerable. There is a weak inscription in body feeling to sustain a sense of self as alive, as capable of self-soothing and of doing well.

As a mother provides care to her child's body-related needs, she inscribes that body with her understanding of what to do, her phantasies, and her desires. In caring for her child, she awakens her child's body into sensitive organic regions called erogenous zones. The work she provides is based on her worldview, her choices, and her tastes. Experiences inscribed in the body form a discontinuity, an otherness, a product of language, which makes it possible to generate images as signifiers that articulate our lack without exhausting it. Unexhausted, we keep working and elaborating.

The representational scripture constitutes one's own body as unique while constituting a subject of desire. In this sense, body image is a mystery and belongs to the unconscious. It is crafted in the historical development of our subjective experience alongside creating the subject. It only becomes preconscious through pain, and as such, is ephemeral (Nasio, 2008).

Once perceptual organs are developed, molded images are added to bodily sensations and their concomitant emotions. Under the sway of the pleasure principle, all that constitutes a source of pleasure is absorbed or "introjected." Whatever raises discomfort is pushed out into the external world or projected. Thus, pleasure principle is not about searching for hedonistic joy. Pleasure involves a level of unpleasant tension.

The newborn is not aware of the external world. A baby lives in a sensory environment that starts by being meaningless. Stimuli impinges upon the baby, as much as the infant acts upon their world. An infant cannot access an object in its totality. At this stage, the child access partial-objects. During the interaction each sense use will provide an experience; but the child cannot add and organize all the information into the creation of one full object. Furthermore, the child cannot differentiate between internal and external realities, between self and object. "A pain in the foot does not immediately draw its attention to the foot, etc. It is rather a wandering pain which is not localized (Piaget, 2013, p. 128). Every action has a concomitant emotion, without discernment between self or other. External realities intertwine with the child's own phantasies as the psychological representative of libidinal desire and aggressiveness that do not originate in articulated knowledge of the external world. Early experiences remain in our unconscious world. Phantasies are like a theater or private world of the self that articulate in a narcissistic way. In his private theater, Mr. Whyte felt people would speak offensively about him.

The total undifferentiated primitive experience is gradually organized into different aspects of experience, as bodily movements, imaginings, knowings, and so on (Isaacs, 1948; Riviere, 1936). In 1912, Henry Head and Gordon Holmes described body schema as the sensory-motor capacity that controls movement and posture. For them, body schema alluded to the representation one makes of one's own body as a volumetric object, as well as its position and configuration in space. This postural model was considered to update itself through movement.

Originally, body schema and body image were two terms used interchangeably. Nacht (1952) illustrated the initial development of body schema as starting at six months of age. This evolution takes place concurrently with the maturation of the pyramidal system and the myelination of the fibers in order for coordination to occur. "It seems that the originally diffuse, incoherent, internal bodily perceptions must first become capable of being consolidated and projected outward in action conducive to the gratification of instinctual needs, before such feeling of unity of the ego can be established" (Nacht, 1952, p. 56).

When I interviewed Dr. Kamala in 2016, she was a petite 65-year-old woman. She used to be a medical doctor in her native country, Sri Lanka. She moved to St. Louis, Missouri as an international student. I met her at her university's library room. She was already waiting for me, albeit my early arrival. She had a generous smile with a slow-paced voice. She took her time to answer the first question. One could tell that she was making an effort to adapt to what she believed I was expecting of her.

On the phone, she told me about her difficulties with her height, being less than five feet tall:

> Initially, when I was young, it did not affect me much. Because of . . . You know, because of my height, I always stood in the front line, sat in the front desk, so it . . . I felt: "Oh, I'm the first." So . . . Uh . . . I was excited about it, but then, later on, as I grew older . . . Uh . . . People sometimes ridiculed me because I was not able to reach up. I always needed a stool. And then, slowly, I started feeling that this is a drawback that I have and it . . . It's not something . . . I'm a below-average height person. So sometimes I used to feel maybe I would not get a good husband. Because in Sri Lanka, we have arranged marriages rather than our own choice marriage. Though I ended having my own choice, but still . . . Uh . . . People used to make comments like that. It . . . It might be difficult. Uh . . . Otherwise, also even when I was in medical college, I used to participate in games a lot but . . . Uh . . . Because of my height, my step was not that

big, so in the long jump, I was obviously never that good. I had difficulty doing the high – um, high jump also. So, these things did affect me, but I would say that maybe . . . I was compensated in other ways. I was always good in studies, so I was appreciated for it. Uh, so people tend to overlook this physical problem. I had a drawback.

Her speech is full of spatial expressions (e.g., look down on, high jump, front line, low marks). Dr. Kamala is a short woman. Being short did not affect her all her life. At the beginning, she felt it to be a positive attribute. Then, one day it became a drawback: "Nobody said it, but it just came to me. I saw others and then I got a bit . . . this inferiority complex in me. . . . It was my inner thoughts, my own thinking that I'm short and I'm not good and all that. That affected me more than what others said. The story is embedded over there and I, whenever I think of it, it's like a pinprick."

Erect position is established during the anal phase. It requires extending the body into the vertical space and mastering the pull of gravity (Kestenberg et al., 1971). There is a certain sense of pride in standing erect and tall, and this is also a value carried by society. Dr. Kamala associates her height with recognition, respect, acceptance, and with cultural practices such as the possibility of a suitable marriage. The fact that she is of "below average" height puts marriage, recognition, and respect at stake. She felt like an "ordinary student." Dr. Kamala appeared to search for talents to feel bright. Her exhibitionistic wish involves showing how smart she can be. This wish operates in the service of self-preservation to compensate for any criticism driven by her drawbacks. She is not tall, lean, and beautiful as her ideal, and the result is an underlying feeling of being "below average."

We have only one body, which is roughly similar through our lifespan. Yet, how we may feel about our body may influence our sense of self, imprint a style of interrelation or, even, disrupt our interactions with the environment. "According to a principle of cognitive economy, there should be a single representation for this unique body. On the other hand, perception and action require different transformations of sensory signals and make different cognitive demands" (Clark, as cited in Pitron, Alsmith, & de Vignemont, 2018, p. 3). While effective action requires detailed spatial content, bodily experiences do not.

Body schema and body image are two concepts regarding enduring properties of the body. Paillard (1999) believes there is a functional duality that fosters the distinction between body schema and body image. Body schema is egocentric and has a sensorimotor function, requiring information about bodily properties for planning and controlling action. Body image is perceptual. It refers to the visual appearance of the body and its surrounding environment. It is allocentric, thus, it can provide information for comparative judgments (Jacob & Jeannerod, 2003).

In body schema, one's own position is taken egocentrically as frame of reference for action planning and executing (Pitron et al., 2018), whereas body image is allocentric. It provides perceptual information about visual appearance of the body and its surroundings. It is discrete, gathering information from social expectations and mirroring practices. It acknowledges the differences between self from others.

Unlike body schemas, the body image is envisaged as available for conscious experience. It possesses an integrated, unified, multimodal character due to the simultaneous representation of visual, tactile, and motor information of corporeal origin (Head & Holmes, as cited in Preester & Knockaert, 2005). Later, Schilder (1935/1950) portrayed body image as the "picture of our own body which we form in our own minds, that is to say the way in which the body appears to ourselves" (p. 11).

Pitron et al.'s (2018) serial model suggests body schema is originally assembled by early multisensory signals of bodily experience. Body schema is earlier than body image. Body image is built upon body schema, but also utilizes diverse sources of information, such as multisensory, mirroring, and social expectations data. Thus, bodily image can be used to adjust body schema. It is more complex, although not as detailed. Body image can be influenced by the sources of information that it utilizes, resulting in a distorted representation, such as in anorexia nervosa. Only body image can acknowledge similarities and differences between self and others (Pitron et al., 2018).

Head and Holmes (1912) highlighted the person's experience of their own body. They used the metaphor of vision being broader than sight. On the contrary, Schilder (1935) described body image as a "picture." Thus, these definitions tend toward pulling apart the body from its image. Without a deep understanding that I am my body, and my body is me . . . and all this does not happen in a vacuum.

For neuro-psychoanalyst Solms (2013), two aspects of the body are represented in the brain. These two aspects are represented in distinctive ways – one internal and the other external. He found that the cortical surface, contains several maps. Each map represents a unique component of somatic sensation (touch, pain, vibration, temperature, etc.). Broadly speaking, body image arises not *in* but *from* these unimodal cortical maps. Mirror neurons activate in the same way whether regarding an object or to the self. "The external body is represented as an object" (Solms, 2013, p. 5) among assorted external objects. The second aspect of the body is internal, autonomic, and barely represented on the cortical surface. These two aspects of body representations are hierarchically organized "bottom-up" and "top-down" to allow the flow of information and appropriate adaptive responses to secure integrity.

Nasio (2008) found three distinctive body images: Stable (biological), functional (full of organic tensions), and the erogenous body image. In his proposition, the sense of self ultimately results from all unconscious body images organized by time and memory. Time finds its origin anaclitically in the rhythm of biological exchanges (Aulagnier, 2015; Sami-Ali, 1990). Space and time are conditions required for the signs of somatic life to become signs of psych life. Later on, they also become the basic elements of our narrative work and social interaction. Body and self need to have some level of development before a child can acquire narrative work skills. The body increasingly articulates itself as a separate object self at the same time as the child integrates and registers the reality and constraints of the external world.

Sami–Ali (1984, 1990) suggested envisioning the body as a space, perfectly interdependent. The body can structure its space by following particular dimensions which are governed by pair of opposites (e.g., inside – outside, high – low, left – right, near – distant, and self – other). Although for Fisher and Cleveland (1968), there is not "a" body image. The construction of a body boundary serves us as a guiding map for self/other interchange. By the end of the second year, the child has acquired a basic sense of ownership over that special space called "I."

By recognizing right from left and so on, a child learns spatial positioning and its particular extensions (e.g., learning to write). The projection of bodily space is ultimately the projection of one's own representational space. "The body involves a paradox: It means simultaneously taking ownership of the body, its desires, and limitations, and integrating the fact that the body is the site where we meet the other, where we negotiate the meaning of sameness and difference, of dependency and separation" (Lemma, 2010, p. 27). It could be said, as Cash and Pruzinsky (2002) did, that body image is a multifaceted psychological experience of embodiment.

For Pankow and Goldstein (1974), the body and its images are supported by two symbolic functions. The fundamental role of body image is the function of unity and gestalt. The second function of body image refers to the ever searching of meaning of the body or its parts. It is my understanding that meaning has the sexual power of reestablishing unity and good gestalt. Being good gestalt an imaginary way of achieving harmony or, as it is called in biology, homeostasis.

The body image, judgments, and a way of being in the world

Although tall, Mr. Whyte appeared rather small, with a somber aura and a bowed back. His entire posture expressing the deep shame he was constantly feeling. Mrs. Clayton described her parents in aggressive terms. She saw herself as monstrous and detestable, resembling the aggression felt through mirroring herself on them. She relayed to me having "no one good memory of her childhood." Negative self images often spring from childhood experiences. It is important to find out what function do these images have. Otherwise the narcissistic gain can turn into therapeutic resistance. These patients are longing for acceptance and friendship. Unfortunately, relationships are highly ambivalent, shaded by fear of losing identity, of being engulfed or being used, as well as many other anxieties.

The word *image* can be traced to the Latin word *imago*, to imitate (Skeat, 1910). In Evans' (1996) *Dictionary of Lacanian Psychoanalysis,* the term is clearly related to 'imago' but "is meant to emphasize the subjective determination of the image; in other words, it includes feelings as well as a visual representation"

(p. 85). For Lacan (1958), vision introduces the central role of desire as a linguistic process. Kristeva (1982) emphasized the presymbolic dimension of the experience (e.g., bodily energies, rhythm) in which meaning is semiotic. "The human body is not an inert object. It is carried, 'worn,' decorated, ignored, experienced. Not only is our exterior – our skin, hair, eyes, teeth, and so on – enculturated, but so is our interior. How deeply we breathe, how we habitually feel about ourselves" (Grimes, 2000, p. 49).

The body is a carrier of messages. Some of them are personal, despite coming from our dealings with family, friends, media, or people we don't know. Some of these messages are like spores or a seed that, with time, can grow into trouble. Like Mrs. Hoocker, a woman with breasts big enough to "hold a six pack," there are women that have breasts so small they don't feel attractive and pursue surgery.

There are noses that are "no-banana" or mouths resembling the Joker's. Our cultural world is full of messages powered and spread by the media. We are not innocent bystanders. We believe those messages and circulate them around or let them go free, unattended, to hurt someone else.

Years ago, a man came to see me with his sign language interpreter. He and his wife were deaf. His in-laws had always been supportive. Now that his wife was hospitalized, he felt they were intrusive and did not know how to handle them. At the end of the session, he felt uncomfortable, and asked me why I had not mentioned his being *oppressed*. He told me that at the institution for the deaf where he attended, he had been alerted of the oppression he would have to accept. Alerted, he was expecting something that did not happen. I had referred to his brother-in-law as being *paternalistic*. After all, the patient acknowledged they had all been truly interested in helping. But they had been doing so with the ignorance of those that act without clear guidance. Life has a different color when we learn to appreciate the acts of kindness (Figure 2.1).

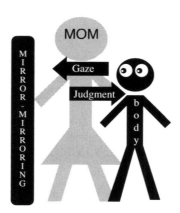

Figure 2.1 Gaze can leave us with a feeling of desecration, wellbeing or grandiosity.

Mrs. Alem was a 60-year-old German participant. She had straight blond hair that fell shortly below her shoulders. Big round eyeglasses covered her blue eyes. She was relaxed as she spoke. Her interview started with an old memory of when she was a child and her mother used to criticize her.

She practiced a mental exercise of looking at a mirror or using others as a mirror to later ponder her own shape. That exercise had a concomitant feeling, which she used in building her own sense of self. As her mother once did, Mrs. Alem believed the need to have a certain look was a requisite to belonging to a given group. If different looks are available, each of them determines relationships and activities or vice versa. She wished to be invited to the parties in the big house but was concerned about not having the appropriate look. Now she owns a company and buys diamonds as a hobby.

> Now when we moved in that new neighborhood where we are now, it was this nice, fancy house. There was, uh . . . appearance's sake I guess, because my neighbors went to a certain gym; they all had their nails done weekly; they all went to the beauty shop every week or three times a week. And I looked that I don't . . . I . . . I guess I could have joined, but I just didn't feel like it. So I guess I didn't quite look like . . . like they felt you look when you're in that neighborhood.

She explained how, as a child, she used to sew herself a nice dress to wear when invited to fancy parties. Once there, she enjoyed herself but felt she was only "visiting," not belonging. When she was young, she could not afford to belong to the lavish group. Later on, once she had a successful business, she still felt like she could not belong to the elite group.

Mrs. Alem described herself as a "tomboy" until her teenage years. She would hang out with her brother, four years her senior, and his friends. She enjoyed skiing downhill, going out for a walk around the lake, climbing trees, or playing soccer and swimming. Around age 16, she became the nicely dressed girl. She attended upscale and high society events through her father's tenure as a professor, all of which appears as the glamour reflected in the magazines she used to read. Leaving behind the "nicely dressed girl," she reincarnated into what she now calls an "athletic woman." Wearing jeans and comfortable shoes is a revamped version of the tomboy she once was. It allowed her to return, in an imaginary way, to her old space of joy and pleasure. Participating in the German Club and the Caféklatsch might have also helped her better connect to that side of her life.

Some terms have the power of drawing up the extension and boundaries of a concept. Body image seems to be equivalent to physical appearance (Jackson, 1987) or physical attractiveness (Feingold & Mazzella, 1998). Reading through the literature generates the impression that emphasizing image results in the body being mostly deemed as a social object. Body image is a site where body, mind, and culture meet (Hutchinson, 1982).

Our mind is the representational device that processes and transforms mental representations. It is not a surprise that Fischer (Fischer and Cleveland, 1968; Fischer, 1986) was unable to prove the existence of "a" single body image. Consequently, it is possible to argue the existence of a dynamic sense of body and synchronic image of it. As synchronic, a child looking at their reflection in the mirror sees themself as whole, whereas the diachronic experience of it is much different. Body image is at times conscious, but it also unconsciously influences how we feel about ourselves and how well equipped we believe we are to deal with our environment, with our friends and family, or with our employers, etc.

The complexity and richness of this concept is well established. However, perception is far more than sight. An emphasis on image, with its own strong visual connotation, could be misleading. Even Lacan (2001) when describing the child's primary identification with the image found on a looking glass, moved away from the primacy of the imaginary and into the symbolic and real registers. An emphasis on the visual could delineate the boundaries of a reality that emphasizes body satisfaction, appearance, and related conceptions as it has in the past. Continuing to do so would leave a few elements, alternative perspectives, and variety of initiatives inconspicuously in the shadows.

3 We are all Zeligs

Participants of the research project revealed having an exhibitionistic drive. I dare say we all have some level of exhibitionistic drive. Most of the time, we seek a glimpse from a meaningful person or from anyone. We want to be recognized. Employees of the month get their picture on the wall. There are those that pay to have their names inscribed in their favorite restaurant, park bench, or walkway.

People tend to look at each other's eyes and "read" their faces, making non-verbal communication possible. In this interaction, there is a look at and a reflection. There is a holding and a taking in, a way of being someone and a way of displaying the self. It is a liminal representation process in which the relation between self and others is put on the table and negotiated. Others are invited to enter the interplay as audience. By playing audience, they are requested to pay attention and to believe. This search for gaze and belonging comes with a price.

In Greek philosophy, "person" is a role someone plays in society. There is no distinction of individuality more than the one involving a place and an inter-role in society. The very instant we ask a child to say "thank you" when they do not feel grateful, we are asking them to develop a social persona apt for social norms even when doing so might require telling a lie. This is not the false self that is described by Winnicott, which is an outcome of rearing. Some people may see social roles as a set of restrictions. Nevertheless, as Sartre suggests, free-dom, the opportunity to be authentic to ourselves, is in the approach we take to make the roles we are given ours. It is in the way we decide to play each part of our lives. Thus, a role is an opportunity and for that we can be grateful.

We are constantly comparing ourselves to others. We keep using people as our personal looking glass and often leave unquestioned what we see about us through them. Unquestioning, we forget the truth lies between the tingle of two different bells. Instead of talking about freedom, we could allow ourselves to freely question the real or imagined messages received. We are concerned, sometimes afraid, that we might not get the expected attention, that we might not be welcome. At one point or another, so many of us feel like we are made out of glass. People see through us or don't have time to look and participate in our lives.

Woody Allen (1983) made an interesting mockumentary called *Zelig*. As a chameleon, Zelig transformed himself to take part in his surroundings. Whatever he thought people wanted of him, he was. He gave each person what he considered they were expecting of him, making sure to connect and receive some sort of recognition from those around him. In this way, he regulated the relationship he had with them and obtained their attention. After all, *selig* means "blessed" in Yiddish.

Using the environment as a frame of reference to his depicted character, Zelig was a Chinese person among the Chinese, an important mobster in a cabaret, a psychiatrist when sent to the hospital, and so on. Camouflage is used to blend in and become one with the surroundings. Masking practice has been ongoing since the Bronze era as a way of bringing out the Other within. For Zelig, masking was mimicry. Ultimately, it was a way of fitting in, of being in harmony with those around him, a form of embodiment by social bonding. The person wearing a mask temporarily ceases to exist in itself to transfigure into the attributes of the mask (Danielsson, 1999). Zelig acquired those traits that turned him into an object of desire. Spectators in the movie actively performed and participated in the ritual, making Zelig difficult to find. Whether he was hiding behind the mask of a Chinese, a mobster, a psychiatrist, and so on.

In the study, those who felt judged by a child thought children do not lie. The innocence of children was remarkable for many participants. They were considered to tell the truth no matter how painful – as if a child held the social aura historically given to the jesters, those fools responsible to bring the most painful of truths to their king. In contrast, if the message was given by a friend, the participant thought that friends would not want to harm them. In other words, nobody questioned the veracity of the judgment. As with Zelig, they just absorbed it – made it happen. Let themselves be transformed by the judgment. Mrs. Teak saw her hands looking as old as her student said. She lost the ability to look at her hands with her own set of eyes. As I said before, maybe the truth lies between the sound of two bells. Having two ears to listen gives us the option to attend outside sources with one, and keep the other ear to listen to the truth our hearts whisper.

Mrs. Clayton has long, skinny legs and blond hair falling on waves over her shoulders. She moves back and forth on the sofa, and her hands do not seem to find rest. As a child, she was repeatedly abused by her father. She described him as a "piece of shit." Then, she said the same thing about herself. She fails to see the beauty I find in her. Her grandmother appears as the only loving figure in her past. She "picked up the slack."

We use more than just our sight to see our face in the mirror. Our sense of self comes from within, but also in accordance with our audience and surroundings, what we have lived through and our expectations for the future. As in the case of Mrs. Clayton, her early mirroring experience, the abuse, and the messages received during her early life have convinced her that she is wicked and worthless. Those messages have stayed echoing in her mind to this day. Every eventuality that she endures is not merely an incident but proof and evidence of her inadequacy. I believe that she is a survivor and that she has played all her cards with one thing in mind – her exert for life. As children do, she believed her parents and became what they saw in her. She felt inept and unable to "pursue a career or do something of herself," as she says.

Melanie Klein (1931/1990) believed the illusion of safety, control, and integration comes from the relationship with the mother's good breast. A child can accept being distant from their mother once they have crafted an object in their mind to maintain the idea of the mother in her absence. Doing so is a way of continuing to feel as safe and integrated as when they are with her. The child cannot maintain self-integration without this trick. It is a trick that repeats again during the mirror stage of development. At this stage, the child looks at the mirror to acquire an image of the self for the second time.[1] They see themselves in the mirror, where they are not. By doing so, the child once again crafts an object that offers constancy and cohesiveness. But this time, as an anaclitic or narcissistic object self, articulating themself as a separate individual. As anaclitic, the qualities are acquired from the attachment figure to continue to gratify their dependent longings. As narcissistic, the qualities are closer to the imagined but unreached ideal. We aspire to meet our perfection and satisfy our narcissistic need for others, because it is the only way to secure our survival (Figure 3.1).

Reciprocity and alliance involve a power struggle that simultaneously defines both the personal and the social. We seek the reflection of our souls in our parents, our mentors, on our friends, peers, neighbors, and employers. At

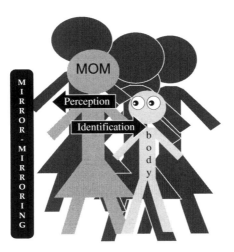

Figure 3.1 The act of perception goes from and to the self, is active and passive. We use others as our looking glass, and we expect them to confirm our sense of wellbeing

minimum we might seek a "hi" from people we do not know but pass by regularly in the coffee shop, the street, or elsewhere. In Lacan's early writings, the mirror stage was an experience happening between six and 18 months of age. He later understood mirroring as structural, as an all-encompassing human tendency. As such, it is considered a phase and not just a stage.

For the French psychoanalytic school, the first and foremost signifier is that of the Name of the Father. A signifier does not only refer to a signified. A signifier is in sequence with other signifiers. It is a process that never ends because "desire is desire for the o/Other" (Lacan, 1971/2009a, p. 425; 1975/2009b, p. 742), "desire is desire for something else" (Lacan, 1971/2009a, p. 175) and "desire is desire for knowledge" (Lacan, 1971/2009a, p. 349; 1975/2009b, p. 764). The unconscious activity of desire is expressed through the associative and combinatory links of the signifier and is repeated in a kind of succession that sets up a chain reaction. Then, meaning is restless, relational, and lays between signifiers. As we create and recreate our persona, we are tirelessly searching for what it means to be us. But meaning can also be fixed when exposed to a frozen signifier (Skelton, 1995). For the French school, the unconscious process of desire is exposed by metaphor and metonymy language processes happening through our utterances, narrative works, and miscellaneous creative acts such as dreams. One can only access the unconscious desire through this articulation.

Since birth we are surrounded by things that come to represent the extension of socio-cultural values. It is a matrix that creates, gives support, names, but also sets restrictions. Early mirroring does not happen in the empty. The looking glass returns a view of all the various items that happen to be on view – among them, a child. How does the child find their own image amid all these things? The first mirroring play is imaginary. It is a continuation of the early exhibitionist unfolding before the mother. The early experience of mirroring in mother's face is an experience of omnipotence and affirmation. A good enough mother offers a sense of vitality, coherence, and competence. The infant first plays in front of a mirror at the imaginary registry, as a sensory alter ego. The child needs to achieve some level of symbolic relation for the mirror stage to properly happen. In front of the mirror, the child is both active and passive, object and subject, and starts to be able to self-regulate.

Cognition is recognition. As if a ray of light had rested on the surface of an entity so that the ego could emerge from the depths. The image found is introjected or incorporated with pleasant feeling. That image offers a setting to the unsymbolized interior, already charged by meaningful impressions, to flourish as a figure on a background. Unsymbolized interior of erogenous zones and bodily organs grumbling turned into action and memory traces that can be articulated. Now the child, having achieved individualization, can also articulate their self as a narrative in the concert of being one other person in the universe. The child enters the symbolic registry and the spatial dimensions to identify themself in the looking glass. All the linguistic constructions come to regulate their identity. They discover what is theirs and what is not.

The toddler first needs to be able to consider the body states perceived from within (i.e., heartbeat, temperature) and the perceptual consciousness of that body seen in the mirror as an ego, being the image their own body image now perceived from another alienated angle. The child recognizes themselves there where they are not, as a subject of desire (Roudinesco, 2006). "Desire is desire for the o/Other" (Lacan, 1975/2009b, p. 425/742). In mother's confirmation of the image, there is a message of belonging. The looking glass has always shown me with my surroundings. I am not just there. I am the effects of the relationship between elements. "What is involved in the triumph of assuming [assomption] the image of one's body in the mirror is the most evanescent of objects, since it only appears there in the margins: The exchange of gazes" (Lacan, 1971/2009a, p. 55). *Assomption* that mother corroborates, letting the child take in the fugacious triumphal phallic role of the symbolic order within the exchange of gazes. Her gaze here supports and confirms the child's discovery. A discovery of their individuality, which means gaining independence and the transformation of the dyadic relationship.

Mrs. Clayton described her mother as someone who never cared about her.

> She is always saying stupid shit. If I tell her I am broke, she just tells me to move on. As a child, my parents used to tell me I was scrap. If I was given a toy to play with, they would take it away and smash it into pieces in front of my eyes.

The reflection on her mother's face, as well as the interaction with both her parents while growing up, failed to support a positive sense of self. She said she was sexually abused by her father. Her mother appears as damaged and damaging. As someone that cannot repair her when she is broken, and breaks her toys when they are intact. Mrs. Clayton is a survivor of the emotionally disturbing environment she had in her childhood.

The looking mirror does not only show a child. It also shows the child's toys, blanket, and all things that are meaningful to the child. For the child, these things are "mine" or they belong to their family. The child is standing in an evocative environment of relationships that are reflected on the mirror as well as is the child. From there, the ego is not only surface and depth, but reflection, reflective practice, and transcendence.

The body is not only an image. It is not just the child looking at an image identified as self, and it is no longer limited to the here and now. That image and that body the child has identified with has a libidinal history. The fetters for those growing up in survivor mode are the strong unhealthy messages. Those messages still echo in Mrs. Clayton's mind, in spite of her no longer living with her parents. Those sadistic messages claim a masochistic gain, which often hinders clinical work.

The body idea is not restricted to the ability to represent it. The child enters into the symbolic registry, turning their body into somatic signs for narrative work within a social domain. A good enough mother undertakes this narrative work in a healthy way for her child. At one point, the child will keep doing this job on their own. The meaningful environment works as a background from where to articulate the meaning of the body and its parts, but also from where to learn what it is to be oneself. Like a surface that needs four legs to make a steady table, the child evolves within an environment into a new level of aware- ness called "I." Finding meaning is using the affective logic to bring back the sense of coherence and unity once felt as omnipotence.

Mrs. Clayton is tall and beautiful in my eyes, but she is broken inside. She fails to see what I see in her. Unfortunately, Mrs. Clayton's self-image is frag- mented and full of wickedness: "I don't feel I deserve the time of the day from people." The early reflections she was exposed to as a child led her to develop an unhealthy self-image. Her sense of self limits her ability to socialize and reduces her level of functioning. She presents a preoccupied–fearful attachment style, characterized by a desire to be liked and accepted by others while fearing rejection and abandonment.

As previously said, it is important to understand that the infant comes from an oceanic experience. Such experience is followed by maternal care that both supports the illusion of the newborn as being all powerful and allows for some controlled level of frustration. Winnicott (1971) said the mother needs to be "good enough" to support her baby's sense of having undisputed sway while still allowing "enough" frustration. That is to say, mother needs to let her infant be exposed to the nuisance of living to incite the development of life skills in her child. Yet, at the same time, the baby needs to be "good enough" to avoid the overflow of frustration on their mother. That is, the baby helps mother deny her lack and sustain her phantasy of wholeness. Remaining with her ensures their being as an object of her desire. Having been born immature, a baby needs to be cared for to endure, grow, and gain appropriate life skills. A moth- er's love allows her to continue to care for her child even under overwhelming frustration and exhaustion. Such care and love ensure her child's survival.

The development of the ego consists in a departure from primary narcissism and gives rise to a vigorous attempt to recover that state. One part of self-regard is primarily the residue of infantile narcissism. Another part arises out of the omnipotence, which is corroborated by experience (the fulfillment of the ego ideal), whilst a third part proceeds from the satisfaction of object-libido. The ego ideal has imposed severe conditions upon the satisfaction of libido through objects; for it causes some of them to be rejected by means of its censor, as being incompatible (Freud, 1914/1953, p. 2954).

For a while and under the sway of pleasure principle, the baby relates to subjective-objects that are under their magical omnipotent control. These sub- jective-objects are narcissistic creations. Every touch or smell. Each sensory experience leaves a pre-symbolic memory trace. These experiences are what Freud called thing-representations. These traces are early organic drive experi- ences of gratification and discharge. Thus, they escape the censorship imposed.

As previously said, the child comes from a state of undifferentiation in which subjective-objects are under their phantazied powerful control. In time, further differentiation and integration takes place with the assistance of a good enough mother (Winnicott, 1965). By then, the child will learn to find the object, recognizing there is a reality that is not under their control. Recognizing object "me" from objects "not me," and moving from omnipotent magical reparation towards a more realistic reparation.

The ego function, its strength, and its health all depend on three aspects of infant and child care: (a) Integration, which matches with the mother's holding of the infant; (b) Personalization, the development of the body ego and of a firm union of ego and body, which depends on the mother's ability to handle the infant; and (c) Object-relating, both to things and persons, which is in relation to the mother's way and timing of object-presentation (Winnicott, 1965).

This is the entrance into the reality principle and the linguistic world. By taking the body as a first object, the ego becomes the central reference point of consciousness.[2] The ego is a coherent organizing entity that manages inner and outer realities. Maternal assistance is the first agent to give signs their meaning, and does so following her own tastes. Narratives usually have three stages: Balance-disruption-balance regained. Narrative work is a way of bestowing reality of certain coherence and good gestalt, despite of losing stability for a while.

For Sophie de Mijolla-Mellor (2005),

> Unlike meaning (signification), which unites a signifier, the material manifestation of the sign, to a signified, the concept to which it corresponds, sense (sens) has an axiological dimension: It is a sense "for" and orders a behavior by linking an object to a desire.
>
> (p. 1021)

Piera Aulagnier (2015) proposed the preverbal infant manifestations of needs are interpreted by the mother as signs that have a sense, and the primacy of affective logic within the dyadic relationship. Once again, having the baby been mother's phallic object, the care she provided - supporting the baby's grandeur - will later spring into an ideal ego for the child.

"The human being has two original sexual objects: Himself and the woman who nurses him" (Freud, 1914/1953, p. 2944). Love feels like being closer to the ideal. It feels closer to the omnipotence and wholeness inherited from primary narcissism and forever aspired to regain. What cannot be regained in reality can be achieved in the metaphoric world of narrative representations we build about and for ourselves.

> Constructing sense makes the I's relationship to reality coherent; such, then, is the primary function of the activity of thinking and, accordingly, delusions themselves will have as their function the creation of a meaningful interpretation of the violence undergone by the subject.
>
> (de Mijolla-Mellor, 2005, p. 1022)

In a story, the hero has the power to successfully overcome the most challenging tribulations. The hero is then the narcissistic aspect of a narrative. A hero's triumph is the positive message against the risk of disintegration anxiety.

Taking the ego as an object does not necessarily negate the other. A child learns to accept, internalize, and speak the discourse of their parents as representative of the big Other. In order to meet their needs and wants, a child learns to recognize the strategy that works with them – a tone of voice, a certain word, or a timely moment. Bodily needs and libidinal economy are denaturalized, subjected to socio-cultural forces, and overwritten by signifiers that exert symbolic Otherness.

To take the ego as an object is choosing the Other as a model, or at least, for good or bad, as part of the equation. Unfortunately, in the case of Mrs. Clayton, this is not pleasant. Her first experiences, the representation she has of her mother, as well as the representation she has of herself are constant sources of suffering.

The relationship with the o/Other is introjected by identification.

> At the very beginning, all the libido is accumulated in the id, while the ego is still in process of formation or is still feeble. The id sends part of this libido out into erotic object-cathexes, whereupon the ego, now grown stronger, tries to get hold of this object-libido and to force itself on the id as a love-object. The narcissism of the ego is thus a secondary one, which has been withdrawn from objects.
>
> (Freud, 1923/1953, p. 3980)

The upshot of turning object-libido into narcissistic-libido is a transformation of a part of the ego into ego ideal. From then on, the ego will be adrift in respect to narcissism. Being adrift generates an intense aspiration to regain it. The child seeks to recover it in this new form of an ego ideal that is unreachable. This maneuver allows the ego to keep its relationship with the object despite the demands of the id. It is a way of reaching an ideal or an image by saying "Look, you can love me too, I am so like the object" (Freud, 1923/1953, p. 3964). Ego character is a precipitate of abandoned object-cathexes that contains the history of object-choices (Figure 3.2).

Freud (1914/1953) described how the premature polymorphous infant at one point takes their own body as a first object called "I," creating the ego. All the erogenous zones are then organized under the primacy of the phallus, as representative of what it is to feel complete. Freud considered that all the erogenous zones fell under the supremacy of a new order by taking the body narcissistically as a first object. Coming across to the reality of a body that is fragmented and uncoordinated, Lacan called it the *corps morcellé*, and Freud called it disorganized erogenous zones. The child finds their image on a mirror and smiles in joy. That image is used in a defensive way.

For Freud, the notion of fragmentation is present as the unorganized erogenous zones and in mother's absences. For Lacan, the emergence of incompleteness arises with the mirror phase as a phantasy of the body-in-pieces. This incompleteness can be seen in clinical practice as loss of boundary or hypochondria. When there is loss of narcissistic identification, or when vulnerability

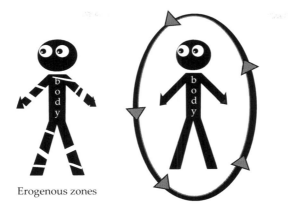

Erogenous zones

Creation of the ego by cathecting the
body as a first object (Freud, 1914/1953)

Figure 3.2 The Freudian description (1914/1953) of the creation of a new structure by
taking the body as a first object goes vis a vis with Lacan's (1975/2009a) account
of the child gaining cohesiveness by identifying with their reflection on the mirror.

is denied by manic defenses (e.g., helicopter ride therapy). The illusion of
omnipotence is a regressive compensatory defense mechanism. Through the
image found in the looking glass, the body gains gestaltic form and gives genesis to the I.

As whatever is pleasant is introjected, the child introjects that image as self. What
is the joy? The joy is to find again the omnipotence they once felt. It is found in an
image that brings a sense of powerful unity. Cognition is the recognition of seeing
one's self complete, which results in a triumphant celebration of someone who had
lost something and finds it again. It is an artifact. It is a way of maintaining integration and continuity in individuation. It is also hope and promise.

Partial drives do not work together; they all find satisfaction in different
erogenous zones, making turbulent movements in the organism and producing the experience of fragmented body. Identification and the reflected image
are used in a defensive way against the vulnerability of the fragmented body,
the increasing level of frustration provided by reality and the increasing distance
from the dyadic relationship that has been maintaining the sense of omnipotence since before birth, which fuels the later narcissism. The identification is
based on sexual and partial drives, and it is highly ambivalent.

As synchronic, that image called I is the inertia of the flesh in its insertion
into the world. It is an image but barely the surface of that image. The image
is taken by sexual drives, bringing a sense of good gestalt. The I is found in
a body that is whole and fully formed. It is not summarized to the sum of its
parts. It is a being. After mother's assertive comment, this image and the sensation that arises remains as an ideal or ego ideal.

Once again, the child recognizes the omnipotence once felt in early narcissism as a possibility and a promise. After experiencing reality as frustrating and castrating, the child recognizes in an image the promise of something that can be achieved again, and that will remain as an unreachable ideal.

Diachronically, there is joy and rage. This rage is the first experience of shame. It is both self-reflective and relational. As relational, the child turns towards their mother and sees her as taller, brighter, better, complete: Perfect. Lacan would call it phallic. The child may feel like caressing the ideal, but what follows is the reality of their limitations. Like an uncanny surprise, self-reflection reminds the child about the body morcellé, and it is a first experience of introjected rage as shame (Figure 3.3).

The I appears as a center at the synchronic level, but the interpretation of such experiences comes from beyond. It comes from our sense of belonging. The I is a subject of language. As diachronic, its horizon is vertical, diacritical, and processed by opposition. The I appears as a center – an outlook for experiences in need of confirmation. It is an aperture as much as it is a repetition. It is vibration and reverberation. Just as the child looks at the image in the looking glass, and looks at the mother, adults trust outside corroboration to be true. The corroboration can come from anyone. Participants believed the messages coming from children as much as they believed the adults, regardless of their understanding of how children and adults had different conceptions of truth and conduct.

Wallon (as cited in Lacan, 1975/2009a) conceived the mirror stage as an entry way into the symbolic order. For Lacan (1975/2009a), the mirror phase is going from the primacy of the imaginary to the reign of the symbolic and the real. The mirror phase involves the use of sight and hearing as gaze. It is not

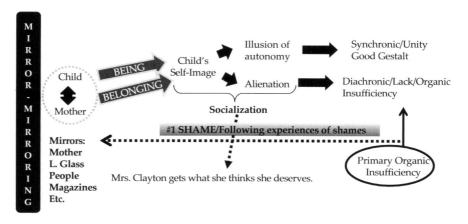

Figure 3.3 The dyad is left behind as the child gains individuality. Mother confirms the image is her child's and sends a message of belonging. The joy is followed by rage. The idealized mother originates a feeling of rage which subsequently appears as shame

visual or auditory per se. Lacan (1980) called it méconnaissance, a misrecognition that represents a certain organization of affirmation and negations the subject is attached to as articulated by desire. Merleau-Ponty (1958) said perceiving is a philosophy, an act of faith. For Lacan (2006) the ego was structured as a symptom due to the arbitrariness of language.

A beam of light clarified the existence of a body for the child. What is hidden on this side of the body gains dimensionality and shines for the world as an I. M/other corroborates the person in the mirror is her child (Lacan, 1975/2009a). This communiqué appears as double binding. It confirms the image captured as being their child's, and in her confirmation sends a message of belonging. It is an endorsement. It encompasses desire of the M/other as an alternative to our helplessness. Image is more than the picture on a looking glass. The imaginary stands to support the illusion that involves a sense of time as promise. Being desirable is at the base of the infant's survival. Indeed, it is at the base of everyone, regardless of their age. The first confirmation of our self-image comes from an idealized Mother. From then on, it will come from idealized Others.

The act of perception goes from and to the self. It is both active and passive. As an interaction with another, there is an expression and a request for love. A mother's face is a primitive mirror in which children learn to see themselves since early infancy. It can result in a positive endorsement or it can be burdensome, as in the case of Mrs. Clayton. Through the mother's expressions and care, a child learns their value and the meaning of all sensed experience they have while growing up. The sense of belonging captures the spatial dimension of their being.

As previously said, from before birth, the child is a receptacle of their parental desires and dreams. The child's body image is exposed to signifiers that follow maternal tastes as well as the libidinal economies of other important people. Hence, the triumph of recognizing that image in the looking glass as the child's ego, as "me," is an act of great courage. It is an act that provides an illusion of autonomy. This private representation of selfhood denies its root; thus, it is a misrecognition. It is also a misrecognition because we identify in the looking glass, where we are not. We take that image as ours, but that image belongs to the looking glass. That image gives us a sense of autonomy, a sense of being who we are.

Mother will confirm the finding by saying things like: *you have your father's smile, and your aunt's nose.* In doing so she is creating a matrix of relationships that sustain our being. Being is belonging. We can never be free if we are to feel safe. Mrs. Clayton's self-image shows how, ultimately, she identified with an image that was an alienating introject she was seduced to accept since childhood. Accepting that image was an act of faith on her part. The image she accepted was the result of her parental conscious and unconscious strategies and maneuverings; of what she is willing to bestow in hopes of being loved.

Mrs. Clayton's masochistic self-critical proclivity has a function – it auspices her negative image. It is an attempt at remaining as the object of her parents' desire. Such is her wish for the most ephemeral gesture of their love. She eagerly awaited most of her life for even a glimpse of positive attention. Later in therapy she was able to recognize her parents do not know how to love them-selves and they are likely unable love anyone else. The moment she accepted she had been waiting for something that might never happen, she started hav-ing more and more positive memories of her childhood. As she said during one of our sessions, her parents were addicted to alcohol and drugs; and she was addicted to her devotion towards them. The risk at that point is repeating such devotion in the therapeutic alliance.

Mrs. Clayton shows us that not all gaze is a healthy holding. One is forever susceptible to the judgments that arrive from the outside world as much as from judgments that come from imagining the self standing in someone else's shoes, seeing from that person's point of view. A mother's holding gaze leaves an impression of safety. Her admiration is a positive value, whereas her disapproval makes her child feel unworthy and expendable and puts their survival in peril (Kestenberg et al., 1971). To preserve the idealized object-mother, the self shuns and a feeling of shame arises. Or, in a narcissistic way, the opposite can happen. The object can be despised as unnecessary in order to preserve the self.

As a survivor, Mrs. Clayton learned to identify with her aggressors and feels undeserving of being with others. "I never feel like I belong. Not even when I am with likeminded people." In the case of Mrs. Clayton, as with so many other people, she wishes she had achieved something in her life. "My school mates all went to college. I didn't. I'm lucky I'm not in jail." She did not attempt to go to college, would not even dare be a professional, and would not look for a good source of income. She has never felt deserving. Like that old saying, she is getting what she thinks she deserves.

We are brought into this world before being fully developed. Our birth happens before we are skillful enough to handle our survival. Belonging, hav-ing someone to behold us, ensures our existence. Even through the mother's absences, a child's sense of belonging evolves with hesitancy along the vicis-situdes of fortune. In the best of cases, at a life-threatening element, the infant cries, a private mother–child language that makes her respond accordingly (e.g., breastfeeding, warmth). The synchronicity of an appropriate action keeps the phantasy of omnipotence going. It is an early experience that marks us for the rest of our lives. It marks how well equipped we feel to handle the inconve-niences we come across. It determines how we feel about ourselves as well as how we relate to our environment and the people we surround ourselves with as we seek to regain our illusion of coherence and mastery. If damaged, it can make us seek signs that corroborate our fragmented, ill, and undeserving sense of self as in the case of Mrs. Clayton.

An infant is perfect, whole, phallic, and an object of desire to their parents. Maternal gaze help sustain this phantasy. Good parental care helps the infant ignore the primary insufficiency of their body. It is an experience that remains unconsciously inscribed, never to be forgotten. It becomes an everyday belief that feeds the narcissism. Without it, facing the challenges of everyday life would be nearly impossible.

Infants are confronted with the truth of their primary insufficiency during the mirror stage. This truth is denied by identifying themself to an image that shows them complete. The child is forever alienated. The libidinal tension then fetters the subject to the endless pursuit of that illusory unity, which is always fading away.

Later in life, it is lived all over again through the mirroring effect that comes from an Other's gaze, shuttering us with the recollection of something we tend to forget – our own insufficiency, which Freud called "castration" and which we experience at times as self-inadequacy. We want to be desired, and our imperfections make us vulnerable. They make us fear not being "good enough" to be desired, again.

On gaze: who is looking at you when you feel you are being watched?

My father spends much of his time sitting by the window in his personal library. A cup of tea (. . . or whiskey) by the side and a book between his hands. Always available. When in trouble or in doubt, coming to my father results in him slowly bringing down the book. His right brow leading the movement of the rest of his face as he prepares to pay attention. The answer to most questions was clear even before uttering a word. Just his look would say it all. . . . Or have these answers always been my attribution? I usually know what he means. I could feel his encouragement, his rage, his preoccupation or respect, whichever applied at the time. No words are ever necessary. I know. I've never doubted it. For him, I am someone worth looking at and that has ever made me more human.

It was interesting to see that regardless of who was judging the participants, the judgment was accepted as true, no questions asked. Forty years ago, a student told his teacher she had old-looking hands. His teacher, Mrs. Teak, was taken by the message. As she processed what she heard, she stopped being a teacher to be captured by the judgment. Ever since, she has been self-conscious about her hands, spending quite a deal of time taking care of or hiding them. Recognizing the body can involve leaving something out, alienated. Mrs. Teak described her hands as a part of her that was somehow apart from her body: "Now that I'm getting old, I'm growing into them."

Through God, St. Augustine does a self-conscious account in his *Confessions* to find himself a sinner. Descartes also used god and discovered the only true thing was his self-awareness, as he expressed as "Cogito, ergo sum." Thus, thought appears to be the principle that rules, even beyond the object world. The primacy of thought invalidates the complexity of our reality. We are also made of flesh and emotion. We live in the time frame of our social world. Yet when we look at those around us, we can see them in their full corporality, not having to deal with the dichotomy of thinking and embodiment. They seem free of such chasms, and we fall prey to idealizing them.

Merleau-Ponty's (1958) concepts usually spring from bodily experience or experience of embodiment. He depicts the act of opening our eyes as a symbol that represents how being-for-oneself implies being-for-others. Being is appearing. For him, self-awareness is going beyond being-for-oneself or being-for-the-other. Self-awareness is a self-reflective practice in which we forget to verify or to judge what we see. Our eyes are no longer perceptive tools for vision. They function under the sway of thought and the spirits in which we are embedded, language being the instrument that precedes us used for such activity. Ultimately, we don't use our sight to perceive, and perceiving becomes an act of faith detached from the world of objects. Mrs. Clayton cannot see herself as beautiful. She avoids mirrors and finds that people loathe her even before uttering a word.

Perception, according to Merleau-Ponty (1958), shows the trueness in things as an act of faith since we have split the world into what is real and what is imaginary. One is the tridimensional social space we create, and the other one is the theater of our personal phantoms. Both influence our perception and understanding. As we come into contact with an object, using our senses and our bodies for perception, we capture the object and that same action affects us. This interplay may leave a positive or negative sensation, inducing disdain or illusion.

What is coherent stands as true and real. But since reality is more likely complex, conflicting, and partial, one would do better by distrusting whatever appears too coherent. Take it as a product of inference rational thinking. Unfortunately, most of us are truth seekers. We want that emotion that dazzles us from believing.

Merleau-Ponty (1958) talked about the frailty of gaze and said that the faith I once had returns to me as skepticism in my being, favoring the Other. One cannot see in others the conflicting dichotomy of body and mind we suffer. We tend to idealize others and find truth in them.

Cooley (1902/1922) considered self-awareness as relational. He regarded selfhood as the product of (real or imagined) judgments we receive from others. His definition is the corollary of three components: (a) the imagination of our appearance to another person, (b) the imagination of a judgment of that appearance, and (c) some sort of self-feeling such as pride or mortification that raises our self-awareness.

Vision makes us feel observant far more than any other perceptual sense, but *looking*, *seeing*, and *gazing* are not the same. Sight is the action of seeing so as to find objects that will ensure self-preservation, according to the reality principle. Gaze is drive ridden. In gaze, there is an excess. Touch and mouth prioritize the sight to increase the area overseen and the success of our survival. Sight and hearing allow us to capture the things of our world from a distance, whereas in gaze there is no distance. Gaze is an intimate experience. In gaze, a sexual drive is satisfied.

"Of course, what most often manifests a look is the convergence of two ocular globes in my direction. But the look will be given just as well on

occasion when there is a rustling of branches, or the sound of a footstep
followed by silence, or the slight opening of a shutter, or a light movement
of a curtain"

(Sartre, 1943/1984, p. 257)

Whether real or imagined, being seen is instrumental, and our bodies make
us vulnerable to other people's judgments. Sartre (1943/1984) presented different vignettes to illustrate reflexive self-consciousness through the lived body
as relational. In Sartre's *Being and Nothingness'* chapter "The Look," gaze is not
neutral. Whether positive or negative, it has an emotional value.

For Sartre (1943/1984), gaze operates by laying a sense of truth upon us.
We are usually in a state of transcendent consciousness. The self is not found in
thought (as Descartes said), but in acts: "My consciousnesses sticks to my acts"
(Sartre, 1943/1984), p. 259). Then by being seen by another, the subject is
reduced to an object. The emotion raised by this experience causes the subject
to separate itself from the activity. Only then do I become visible to myself.
"The Other teaches me who I am" (Sartre, 1943/1984, p. 274). Sartre's gaze
is both ontological and phenomenological. We are in a state of transcendent
consciousness until, through the gaze, we gain both consciousness of the relational status of our being and self-consciousness. It is an embodied experience
that results in a self-feeling.

Sartre's (1943/1984) shame feeling goes past any physiological quality: "I
am ashamed of myself as I appear to the Other" (p. 222). The Other medi-
ates our self-reflective acts. In our transcendental life, we think of ourselves as
wholly and perfect. Shame is a feeling that raises the awareness of the denied
limitations imposed by our bodies and from being a product of language. The
superego utilizes the scopic drive to keep watch of the actions and intentions
of the ego to judge and censor them.

Sartre (1943/1984) said that we are nothing but an object of interest to
another person. All the things of the world revolve around this main person:
The subject. My self-consciousness is present insofar as I am an object for
the Other. All the freedom of my possibilities are reduced to the probabili-
ties given by the situation at hand. For the first time and for the split of a
moment, I am. Sartre said "I am seated" (Sartre, 1943/1984, p. 262). For
Sartre, to apprehend the gaze is to be aware of being looked at, an act that
objectifies us.

I would argue that for a stream of a moment, I escape all possible causal relations and become one self to myself. In such level of abstract self-consciousness,
I can no longer be trapped by the relations that make of me an object for the
Other. By becoming aware of my consciousness, I vanish. Self-consciousness
has an aphanisis effect on the object I was when the Other stared at me. I was
an object for an Other, but the moment I gain self-consciousness, I become
my own center. I am detached of all causal relationships. If the Other is still
looking at me, my awareness is no longer weighing His will. It was His gaze
that pulled me out and away.

I accessed the loneliness of my being, and it was terrifying. Out of any relation, there is no possible life. That is the jouissance. Eros brought me back into the world. Scared, I place my eyes on the path of the drive in their return from the Other, bringing back an effect as if the Other had placed judgment on me. I accept (. . . or resent?) the Other's gaze because it makes me feel securely tight into the world. I welcome it. I can breathe once again. Attached to this world, for good or bad, I am alive.

It is a terrifying experience to access the loneliness of my being in that way. Uncanny, Freud would say. In *Instincts and Their Vicissitudes*, Freud (1924/1953) marks the three tempos of the scopic drive: An early satisfaction in the body through an erotic zone, a search for an object to "compare with," and finally the return to the self. Following the antithetical voyeurism-exhibitionism, sadism–masochism, active–passive, Freud noted our narcissistic taking of the body (Other's/one's own body) as an object. Another object is looked up (voyeur) for the satisfaction of sadistic drives. In doing so, the subject utilizes that other person as a way of seeing themself. As the body is taken narcissistically as an object, both self and other are co-constructed. We wish to be whole and to feel connected.

One of the earliest descriptions done by Lacan (1981) in reference to the gaze was of an episode he had one day when he went out fishing:

> I was on a small boat with a few people from a family of fishermen. . . . as we were waiting for the moment to pull in the nets, an individual known as Petit-Jean . . . pointed out to me something floating on the surface of the waves. It was a small can, a sardine can . . . It glittered in the sun. And Petit-Jean said to me – Can you see that? Do you see it? Well it doesn't see you.
>
> (p. 95)

For Lacan, gaze is a drive expression of our desire. It makes evident our castration. For Sartre, gaze is a binary dialectic relationship subject–object/master–slave. In late Lacan, the ego unfolds in moi and I, turning the gaze into a relationship between three elements: The Other, object (moi), and subject (I). In the example, the gaze comes from the Other – the can-, which turns him into an object. As a subject, Lacan is the I of a representation. But in the imaginary registry, he can also identify with that person looking at him being looked at.

The "gleam of light" from where the gaze is coming is the place where I imagine the Other is standing when looking at me. Lacan sees himself where he is not. As a subject, he is a representation, a picture. From the point of view of the can, he is the Other, which would turn him into an object. But he is also the subject looking at himself being looked at. In the imaginary registry, there is an identification with that other that is me. The scopic drive takes the body as an object with the pleasant surprise of seeing it as a "picture" I identify with;

followed by shame by eruption of the real. Shame is only registered in relation to an other (Lacan, 1981).

There is a glow of light that transfigures and gives shape to that, which we could otherwise not see. It brightens, veils and reveals. It masks the real. It makes it accessible and tempers it. Without its veils the real strikes.

For Lacan (1981), his story shows a disruption. It is a point of failure "governed" by the "function of the stain." A short-circuit that all together interrupts and produces the experience of the gaze in which the subject fails to see what is really in front of their eyes. They see what the gaze brings up, and the uncanny experience unfolds: "I see myself seeing myself" (Lacan, 1981). For Freud (1919/1953) considers the anxiety we feel at the uncanny is the return of the repressed and marks the existence of our castration. For Lacan, through the gaze the real "surprises us," comes to "disrupt us." By coming across "the lack" we are reduced to a shame feeling that is nothing else than castration anxiety (Lacan, 1981).

For Lacan (1981) there is a tight relationship between the *object petit a* and the gaze. From 1963, Lacan considered *object petit a* as the object that sets desire in motion, particularly in relation to the partial objects that define the drives that find satisfaction through the path by circling around it. At the center of desire there is a lack, which we cover with the screen of our narcissistic projections, and all the social and linguistic constructions that come to regulate our identities. The gaze threatens the eruption of the real, showing that behind our desire there is a lack. Thus, gaze not only sees but also shows. That is the jouissance.

The ego, Freud would say, is confronted with the truth of castration. We are confronted with the truth of our lack, in Lacan's terms. The Other fails to hold us, and we feel as if they would have become the object of judgment. Self-consciousness is looking at myself to find out my denied organic insufficiency and my dependency on others.

Notes

1 The first image is found on their mother's face.
2 For neuro-psychoanalysis the ego is mostly unconscious.

4   Branded by shame, taste values

The body is the vantage point of our existence, and the experience of belonging to a body is our sense of self. Body and identity are both personally and socially constructed. Charles Horton Cooley (1902/1922) suggested that selfhood is the result of the imagination of our appearance to other people, the imagination of their judgment of that appearance, and some sort of self-feeling, such as pride or mortification, that arises from that judgment. I'm suggesting such feeling of mortification is shame. I'm also suggesting that shame follows a logic of sacrifice as defensive mechanism, which is based on taste values. Sacrifice is a private cleansing tribute that helps transfigure into something acceptable and of higher grounds.

Appearance

The research I performed started with the prompt, "Have you ever been praised or criticized about your body or any part of it?" It was not difficult to find participants. Most of them had a particularly sensitive part of their body for which they've suffered most of their life. Dr. Dillon took his shirt off on a summer day when he was about 14 years old. He's never done that since. Now he is in his fifties and continues to avoid going to places where he is expected to take his shirt off.

There can be more than one sensitive body part. Nevertheless, in this research, participants showed that their particular body part was gravitational to their sense of self. How they felt about themselves, what they did or did not do. . . . it was all somehow an expression of their own strategies to manage the body part they were concerned about and their wish to be accepted by others.

There is a meaning ascribed to judgments. The situation is very well described by Sartre (1943/1984) in occasion of a stroll he took by the park. He felt someone was looking at him. The result was that Sartre gained self-consciousness. It was like a trick to look reflectively back at himself through this other person. He then experienced an emotion regarding his appearance to another person, as if he had been judged by the onlooker.

Sartre (1943/1984) realized it is not necessary to have someone's set of eyes looking at us for this to happen. It can very well be the sound of steps, of a curtain moving. Whereas Lacan (1981) felt looked at by a can. This is what Cooley (1902/1922) mentioned as a gaze raising some sort of self-feeling, whether pride or mortification. A self-feeling that comes out of a real or imagined judgment is the criterion for classification in which we are given the thumbs up or the thumbs down.

Skeat (1910) said to criticize is to discern or to judge following a criterion, as when we are classifying. Therefore, classifying is neither good nor bad, just a way of organizing our experience and our world. Merleau-Ponty (1958) described how we perceive the world with and through our bodies and how doing so changes us.

The sense of who we are is centered upon the body. Self-concept goes shifting through the years as the body develops from childhood and into adulthood. A person can experience change after a broken limb, a scar, or another accidental new body condition. Accordingly, a person can search for change through cosmetic surgery, dieting, or exercising. In both cases, the alterations are not strictly physical. They often have emotional, economic, and social after effects. Furthermore, in order to reach an aesthetic ideal, people follow clothing fashions, wear make-up, and go on a diet or under the scalpel.

Mr. Horowitz's nose was "broken over 25 times. It got in the way. It was that big. It had to get hit." A distinction could be made between an attack upon the ego (a psychic structure) and an attack against the body-self. Both are self-destructive behaviors. Yet, an outbreak against the body may reflect a conflict between ego and superego structures, and it is masochistic. That "it had to" suggests the works of a masochistic superego.

Until the rhinoplasty surgery, Mr. Horowitz's nose carried all the negative connotations a big nose like his could have. The self finds its foundation in the body. Those negative traits turned Mr. Horowitz into something he despised being. Mr. Horowitz identified with his nose. Such identification suggests attacking his body was also an assault against his sense of self.

"I think I told the guy I wanted a pug nose. If I was gonna fix it, I wanted to get rid of it," shared Mr. Horowitz. Then he added that after the surgery, "it was gone: I looked normal."

For Mrs. Hoocker, her breasts appeared as center of attention and gateway with her social surroundings. She kept a safe distance from "dirty old men" and felt people made comments and wanted to touch her breasts to see if they were real. She was known for the size of her breasts. She tried her best to hide her ample bosom between her arms.

Mrs. Hoocker alluded to her breasts in proper, educated terms, as a way of handling the feeling they evoked in her. She used a variety of defensive strategies to manage what this part of her body meant to her. She alluded to the social implications and life events she encountered because of having DDD-size breasts. Her narrative ends with her undergoing reduction surgery, as if her suffering had somehow stopped. I would say her suffering continues at a different level, as illustrated by her showing me the breasts that were not there the first time we met. This was an unexpected finding on my research which I call shadow limb, analogous to phantom limb syndrome. That is, whether surgically repaired or otherwise corrected, the old body part appears in the participants' narratives in the present tense as if it were still active even after repair. I called it *shadow limb* because of its effect on the sense of self of the participants.

There has been a variation on the idealized body attributes throughout history. For Grogan (1999) in the 1970s, slimness came to represent unconventionality, freedom, youthfulness, and a ticket to the "Jet Set" life, and was adopted as the ideal by women of all social classes. "Virtue is nothing but inward beauty, and beauty is nothing but outwards virtue" (Bacon, 1626/2014). Beauty is something to be worshipped as a sacred thing. It has been associated with ideals of truth, goodness, love, and the divine.

Accordingly, evil was thought to manifest itself through frightful unattractive features. Ugliness is the moral opposite of beauty. As early as the first century A.D. in Egypt, prisoners underwent amputation of their noses (Santoni-Rugiu & Sykes, 2007). The cephalic index would visibly express the social, economic, intellectual, and moral undeveloped human sapiens destined from birth to be despicable.

The Greeks, who were apparently strong on visual aids, originated the term *stigma* to refer to bodily signs designed to expose something unusual and bad about someone's moral status. Cut markings or burnt branding the body are some of the ways of advertising the status of bearer as slave, criminal, a traitor – a blemished person, ritually polluted, to be avoided, especially in public places (Goffman, 1963).

Ugly and poor laws regulating appearance have passed in various countries. In the United Kingdom, these laws were passed in 1729 and remained effective until 2004 in the city of Camden (Schweik, 2009). In the United States, the first city to pass an Ugly and Poor Law was San Francisco in 1867, which established that "if any crippled, maimed, or deformed person shall beg upon the streets or in any public place, they shall upon conviction thereof before the Police Court, be fined not less than five dollars nor more than one hundred dollars" (Schweik, 2009, p. 291), $80 to $1,600 in today's money. New Orleans, Louisiana followed in 1883. By 1881, the law passed in Portland, Oregon. Portland's fine was between $560 and $5,600 in today's money (Hume, 1892). Chicago, Denver, Reno, Los Angeles, and other cities followed this trend. Some went as far as including up to six months of jail time, others included fines as little as $1 (equal to $28) for each offense. Even though these laws or regulations were repealed in the 1970s, signs deposing beggars can still be found as close as in my neighbor's house.

Untouchables existed historically in many different countries. The most well-known is the isolation of the leper. France had the untouchable Cagots. The Hindu caste system had the Dalits. In Japan, the Buraku. The "untouchables" comprised the lowest social class. Even after passing laws against untouchability, many of these people remain regularly outcasts. Different justifications make them untouchable, such as being in contact with desecrated specimens, in charge of death-related tasks, or exposed to wicked forces.

Ugliness is not limited to aesthetics. Someone can face ostracism by expressing an idea considered antiestablishment. When I was a graduate student at Washington University in St. Louis, I refused to submit to the university's use of my $5 student group fee to fund hurricane Katrina relief. I remember clearly how those standing by me walked away as I spoke up, saying social workers should not make donations. In my view, it made far more sense to run a fundraising campaign to create a disaster relief trust fund for all these occasions. After all, several other natural catastrophes occurred around the world that same week, and over 40% of the student body were international students.

A picture from that day shows me totally isolated, as the rest of the students crumbled up at the opposite corner of the conference room. The dean called me up to his office the next day. He had met with the University Chancellor to create a disaster relief fund for all students dealing with this issue back home. The dean never made public that my idea had been accepted by the university, even when a matching fundraising meter was put on display within 24 hours. Touch – and the untouchable – can be symbolic or physical. There is a contagious risk in touching the rejected.

In the *Origin of Species*, Darwin (2018) utilized Herbert Spencer's theory of evolution as the struggle of the fittest. Aesthetics has been what separates lesser developed human beings from those who have achieved higher rank. Beauty is associated with wisdom and rational thinking as opposed to the impulsivity of animals that strive for survival. Indeed, throughout history, attractiveness has been a measurement of virtue. Ultimately, Bourdieu (1984) articulated it in the following terms:

> In a sense, one can say that the capacity to see (voir) is a function of the knowledge (savoir), or concepts, that is, the words, that are available to name visible things, and which are, as it were, programs for perception. A work of art has meaning and interest only for someone who possesses the cultural competence, that is, the code, into which it is encoded.
>
> (p. 2)

For Bourdieu (1984), those who are trying to meet their basic needs of survival can value physical or abstract goods based on practical use, while those who have their needs met have the capacity to find worth by what things represent in the concert of intellectual universe. Thus, the ugly are associated with the criminal and stupid, which is an example of what Marx (1932/2014) called the "animalization of the proletariat." They are less likely to move up in the world. They are less likely to successfully survive the social universe in Darwinian terms.

Appearances matter. The sense of who we are is centered upon how we sense our body looks to others and centers on how we feel about our body. Appearances have been manipulated since early times; for instance, to state social status (e.g., Cappa Magna, especially when using fine elaborated materials) or express opposition to social conventions (e.g., Punks' use of dog collars, swastika, hair-style, tattoos, body modification, etc.).

We don't just have a body. We are embodied in the particular way we use our senses; in the way we dress, walk, or breathe; in the way we look *at* things and interact with the world. In any interpersonal tension, there is someone looking, someone who is on display and someone making an effort to catch a glimpse of another person's gaze, which brings up self-consciousness or makes us feel alive. In every interaction, there is a negotiation. The ugly is repulsive. It is not lovable. It is shunted, whereas beauty attracts, feels welcoming, and creates a group feeling. Our need for social interaction is at the base of our survival instinct. It is required to meet our needs and to feel protected.[1] Our characteristics as an individual not only come from within, but are developed and enhanced by an appropriate social surrounding. What is ugly and the beauty is culturally determined.

Dr. Dillon yearned to feel "integrated" and "protected." At one point in his life, he was accepted as a member of a hostile bully group. "Because I had insecurities, you know, with my limping. I had insecurities. . . . And these bullies would protect you." He did not realize at the time that being a member of this group meant doing things he would not be proud of (e.g., bringing a girl's panties down).

People not only live within a group but also in contrast to other groups or social conventions.[2] For admittance into a group, certain referential codes are required of the individual. Motivated business people from Wall Street wear a special jacket at work. Those jackets mark who they are and who they work for. Professional golfers also have jackets indicating who they are within the golfers' jamboree. In the social imaginary, punks know more about motorcycles than they do about the stock market or golf. We don't expect to find a punk working at Wall Street. Their jackets are made of leather, not of fine fabrics.

Beauty is the variety of qualities for effective attractiveness and alliance. Some groups value relationships over education and knowledge, sports over language skills. There are countless of idiosyncrasies to define someone's personal merits.

Winnicott (1965) suggested that in order to gain independence, the adolescent needed to challenge and dethrone their father. The search for personal identity is also a search for freedom. Group identity is no different. Hippies fought against the power of money with flower power. Punks stood for anti-establishment views and freedom. For the most part, male and female bodies symbolize their gender identities in mutually opposed ways. The search for gender identity beyond the binary has been in expansion – for instance, since the 1980s, with Boy George's cross dressing, Michael Jackson's androgyny, and Annie Lennox's transvestite look.

Choices are made in opposition to those made by other classes (Bourdieu, 1984). By consuming the peripherally transgressive, we acknowledge our differences with others and nourish our psychological self. In this process, there is a confirmation of things ("the other" vs. us; "the other" vs. me). It is before the other that we gain self-consciousness. But there are different ways of relating to that other. Eradicating the master does not make everybody equal. The elimination of the master is the downfall of its slave. In both cases, it is a form of self-eradication.

The social symbolic supplies the transgressors an abject with what strengthen its base of exchange, its status quo, its logic. This abject provides a negative feeling that instills horror while purifying. "Prohibition and transgression – pollution and purification – are, then, tied to abjection. The one who commits an act of defilement feels wretch and worthless" (Lechte, 2003, p. 10). Feeling worthless, they seek being seen. They seek a place or a group of like-minded people who can offer pillar and platform. Eventually, the transgressor signals the existence of a new market. Companies use this new market for their benefit. They call in advertising companies, which broaden the market, increasing sales as the last call in fashion. After each group transgression, and almost without realizing it, the social world ends up accommodating. Sooner or later places alternate and the peripheral becomes fashion and center. The cycle starts again each time a new generation tries to establish their own identity by dethroning the establishment. Winnicott (1965) described it as part of the process of growing up.

In an economy full of disposable objects, objects for one-off use, men and women get the message. The one-off use practice ends up including other human beings. Participants felt at risk of rejection for having body traits that did not conform with today's fashionable looks. Cast-off, they are disposable.

Furthermore, the old body part of those participants who had it healed or surgically repaired appeared in their narratives in the present tense. They were still attending to that special body part. When a part of the body is removed, continuing to feel its presence is called phantom limb syndrome. Participants' narratives expressed a continued presence of the attribute and body parts as a shadow. I'm using the term "shadow" following Freud's (1917/1953) article "Mourning and Melancholia." "Thus, the shadow of the object fell upon the ego" (p. 3047). Participants' repaired body part remained present after surgery, shadowing their freedom from it.

Mr. Horowitz refers to his new nose in past tense: "It was thinner than it is now." His old nose is peeking back at him. Mrs. Hoocker opens her blouse to show me her bosom, the place that confined something that is gone, yet lingers. The representation of their bodies, the unconscious body image, persisted unchanged after reconditioning. While these participants could consciously know they looked "normal," they all had memories and experiences of having lived with a meaningful body part. Repairing the body does not recondition the unconscious image of it. Mr. Horowitz feels more confident with his new nose as a fetish that covers his fault. His concerns of being rejected, the risk of rejection, diminished. He is now a successful businessman out of "small town." His new nose appears to have had a fetish effect. Surgery cannot erase from the unconscious body image once was.

Social ideals of beauty are not set in stone. There is a *zeitgeist* as well as a geographic cultural dispersion in which people don't only speak different slang or languages but, what is possibly more important, inhabit different sensory worlds. Thus, the ideas of beauty and virtue differ. They are constantly being reformulated and transmitted through four essential agents: Parents, peers, as well as the media and the market. Parents can influence directly or indirectly. Direct influence is done through comments regarding body shape, weight, food rules, or comments regarding loss of social desirability. Indirect ways involve unintended parental modeling of their own weight and dieting concerns. Peers can influence through comments or teasing regarding body shape or weight, perceived norms of engagement in peer groups, and the belief that popularity is conditional to one's compliance with a given ideal.

Mass media such as children's toys, fashion magazines, software games, movies, and music videos are considered the most pervasive transmitter of sociocultural ideals of beauty, no matter what gender. For instance, studies found that the more time men and women reported watching television, the higher their reported drive for muscularity (Boyce, Kuijer, & Gleaves, 2013). The Internet is another readily available source of influence showing celebrity sites as well as "pro-ana" (anorexia) sites.

The world is a container of disposable, one-use objects; men and women get the message, or they are trained the hard way. The internalization of body ideals has been related to body dissatisfaction, psychological suffering, and concerns of social desirability in people.

Being protecting or a good breadwinner used to be male ideals. Men at the time did not present as much body dissatisfaction as they did once ideals shifted to body related parameters. As Perloff (2014) pointed out, social media working via negative social comparisons and peer normative processes can significantly influence body image concerns. Yet the relationship between media, sociocultural influences, and body dissatisfaction continues to be complex, multiply determined, and bidirectional. Ultimately, the internalization of body ideals is powered by a wish to belong.

Judgment

The concept of judgment is often used but not well defined in psychoanalysis. Skeats (1910) defined the word *judge* as an arbitrator, which as a role, relies on an array of ego capacities and functions such as memory, mobility, attention, searching, or scanning of the outer world (Money-Kyrle, 1978). Judgment could then be defined as acknowledging the existence of a quality or an object. It springs from reality-testing acts following identity of thought. It is a process of differentiating what is unreal, merely a presentation and subjective and only internal, from what is real; as well as the constant exercise of taking in and putting out (Hartmann, 1956).

Judgment is a function concerned with whether a thing is desirable, or whether it is real. If it is true or false. That which is desirable can be a product of our mind and thus false. It belongs to the pleasure principle. On the contrary, a product of the natural and social realms is usually considered true, but we cannot access it directly. It can be of use for our survival and therefore corresponds to the reality principle.

The pleasure principle is always present, but mental processes used to secure satisfaction (e.g., perception, memory, judgment) are under the sway of the reality principle. So, what is real? Reality is a construction. Thus, as in the case I just described, reality can have different outlooks. In psychology, there is no truth other than the one spoken by (and beyond) the subject, the truth of the unconscious. Judgment operates within a cultural milieu that gives discernment its character.

The reality principle requires capacity for delay of pleasure and toleration of unpleasure. Pleasurable and unpleasurable conscious feelings are attached to the ego and evolve parallel with mental development. The balance of pleasure-unpleasure considers elements directly involved in the present activity and those who await in the future, as so happens especially after the superego has been established (Hartmann, 1956).

In maturing, the child moves away from the mandate of the pleasure principle. This procedure starts with the maternal assistance, who is the infant's first decoder of the world. Mother's wisdom, wishes, and dreams, her savoir-faire, availability, as well as her maternal skills guide appropriate actions in the care of her child. I call all of these her taste values.

From early on, judgments are part of learning successful adaptation. The child thrives and develops with her as a framework. The care mother received as an infant, her cultural domain, her attitude and skills, wishes and expectations all transpire as the taste values she has for her child. They become the framework of affective logic. The origin from where body image blossoms. Mother is the first interpreter, and judgments are at the basis of our survival. "It is really the pleasure principle that gives this move its power" (Hartmann, 1956, p. 38).

From the start, judgments are not only about data but mostly in regard to values. Furthermore, as Buytendijk put it, "one's world . . . is no system of objective correlations, but a system of meanings and thus of values" (as cited in Hartmann, 1956). Emotional values are influenced by social conventions but do not necessarily refer to subject-object relations in the same way. The judgment's emotional value bothered participants of this research, raising self-consciousness and shame. The consequence of moral-rational judgments is guilt, which indicates the presence of the superego. Erikson (1980) placed guilt at the phallic stage and shame at the earlier anal stage, whereas shame responds to affective logic.

For Plato, Merleau-Ponty, Freud, and so many others, we are detached from the world of objects. Plato referred to the idea, Merleau-Ponty to the philosophers, Freud used the word *representation*, and so on. We can only access corporeal experiences rendered into thought and language, which are charged with emotions. The quality could be a property of the item. But when we return to look at it again, it may look and feel different. It may even look back at us and make us different, as so happened with Lacan's (1981) can. We don't use just our vision to access the properties of something that is "out there." We use our mind and corporeal experience, our unconscious wishes or beliefs, and all the elements that might influence us at the moment we rest our eyes and soul to look at something. Whatever it was, it is not found outside but in the between and betwixt.[3] For as we interact, we accommodate and adapt, to borrow Piaget's (1979b) wording. We do not adapt and accommodate just to the object we are holding but to a social order that encircles and sustains us. Taste is an emotional value for the self that is influenced by a social network and powered by desire.

Merleau-Ponty (1958) reminded us that we wrap the object with our flesh every time we take a peek at it. On how many occasions do we mentally savor an ice cream before finding it in the freezer? The acquisition of language opens the child's door to the social world and eventually to thinking instead of acting.

In Piaget's (1979a) theory, the successful action of having sated hunger following the first breastfeeding is what mobilizes a child to repeat the action. Sullivan (1953) asserted that with time, a child learns to judge the existence of good-breasts, bad-breasts, and wrong-breasts. A child will seek the good breast, for the bad breast brings anxiety and the wrong breast requires exhausting work often followed by frustration. Not all knowledge comes from trial and error. Much of our reality is the result of social conventions that are introduced by our parents, peers, and the media. These are among the many lenses used to discern what is perceived and to find meaning.

A mother's face is a primitive mirror in which a child first learns to see the self. Later, the child will look at themself in the mirror. M/other confirms that the person in the mirror is her child (Lacan, 1977). This appears as double binding. A child captures that image as being themself, as integral and independent. In her confirmation, M/other also sends a message of belonging. A child then feels at ease and protected.

Every person wants to be loved and to have that connection. There is a search for that primitive statement of acceptance enjoyed with the first successful object relation. The act of perception goes from and to the self. It is both active and passive. As an interaction with another, there is an expression and a request. The one on view stands as an object of representation in the way they eat, breathe, and talk. They are members of a society and represent their social class (in ethnic, religious, and professional preferences) as well as those more susceptible personal choices such as fashion. One is forever susceptible to the judgments that arrive from the outside world.

But those judgments do not just come from outside. It is not necessary for others to actively judge our appearance. Only our assumption of people engaging in a judgmental attitude towards our appearance could affect our sense of self and how we feel about our body. Head and Holmes (1912) originally described body image as the representation one makes of one's own body as a volumetric object to control movement and posture as well as the body's position and configuration in space. It is not only a personal biological fact. Body image is intrinsically social as well. The image Mrs. Clayton had of her body differed from the way I saw her body.

Piaget (1979b) considered the newborn not to be aware of their body. During the sensory-motor stage, intelligence leads to the construction of an objective universe. Yet the body still appears as an element among others (Piaget, 1979b; Schilder, 1935/2014; Solms, 2013). For Kant (1790/2012), we are conscious of space only to the extent that we represent objects in it; among those objects is our own body. Therefore, subjective judgments of perception are parasitic on objectively valid judgments of experience. Self-consciousness requires that I place myself in an objective world and refer at least some of my representations to objects distinct from me.

Kant (1790/2012) thought of judgment as a very special cognitive power. Judgments don't refer to concepts or ideas of any particular object. It is a practical principle to help us understand and investigate nature. In the *Critique of Judgment,* Kant asked if such cognitive power has a principle of its own. The answer is yes:

> Judgment does in fact have a unique principle and that it is "constitutive," that is, normative, for the feeling of pleasure and displeasure. Moreover, as normative or "rule giving" for this feeling, the principle of judgment is precisely a principle of taste, understood as a capacity to judge or discriminate by means of this feeling.
>
> (Allison, 2001, p. 4)

For Kant, judgments of taste are essentially subjective or based on our own gratifying experience. Judgment's normativity come from the normativity of feeling, which he describes as follows:

> When a man puts a thing on a pedestal and calls it beautiful, he demands the same delight from others. He judges not merely for himself, but for all men, and then speaks of beauty as if it were a property of things. Thus he says that the *thing* is beautiful; and it is not as if he counts on others agreeing with him in his judgment of liking owing to his having found them in such agreement on a number of occasions, but he *demands* this agreement of them. He blames them if they judge differently, and denies them taste, which he still requires of them as something they ought to have; and to this extent it is not open to men to say: Everyone has his own taste. This would be equivalent to saying that there is no such thing as taste, e.g., no aesthetic judgment capable of making a rightful claim upon the assent of all men.
>
> (Kant 1790/2012, p. 52)

In taste judgments, we demand agreement from our audience. Then, judgment reflects more than an individual preference. In matters of taste and beauty, we expect a judgment to be shared. For Kant (1790/2012), judgments of taste aspire to have universal validity: "The thing is beautiful." Beauty presents itself as a property of thing. Kant would call judgment of the agreeable to those who profess relativism. The agreeable judge preaches tolerance but eventually puts their judgments as a measure beyond criticism. If they can never go wrong, then they are like the man who places something on a pedestal for all to agree with him. If the thing is beautiful, it is a property of the thing itself.

Yet, the man could have been expressing his feelings in a genuine way. An erratic judgment, therefore, would be a revealing telltale about the judge and cause conflict. Since taste judgments are normative so long as they are rooted in our cognitive faculties, or – more Kant appropriate – in our capacity for imagination, then, as Bourdieu (1984) did, we could argue that no judgment of taste is innocent. Aesthetic experience and understanding ultimately require holding some type of decoding artifice. Doing so implies a symbolic system as well as a system of power relations. For Bourdieu, taste values are influenced by social conventions. As a telltale sign, something is revealed about the judge through their own ruling.

Taste judgments hatch feelings of shame concurrently with self-consciousness. Sartre said in shame "a part of the self is revealed to the self" (as cited in Schneider, 1992, p. 25). The man who puts a thing on a pedestal and finds that others don't agree with him is likely to endure the uncomfortable feeling of mortification. The uncanny discovery confronts him with the reality of his crime and the horror of finding that he is not up to par. This is especially the case when ruling over something as personal as the body, or a part of it. It is before the Other that one gains self-consciousness. "Through shame I have discovered an aspect of my being. Shame therefore realizes an intimate relation of myself to myself. I am ashamed of what I am" (Sartre, 1943/1984, p. 301).

"I looked in the mirror, and was horror-struck because I did not recognize myself. In the place where I was standing, with that persistent romantic elation in me, as if I were a favored fortunate person, to whom everything was possible, I saw a stranger, a little, pitiable, hideous figure, and a face that became, as I stared at it, painful and blushing with shame" (Goffman, 1963, p. 19).

Value: feeling of mortification

People use visibility as one of the means of performing and presenting identities. People engage in self-presentation within a set of culturally defined hierarchies. These practice positions put people in a pecking order according to how particular aspects of their appearance such as size, shape, and skin quality fit against what is regarded as socially desirable.

Mrs. Clayton craves having friends and feels nobody wants to be with her. She invited someone out to dinner and paid for it. Then she described the experience as "boring. I hate listening to his uneventful life. Why do I have to babysit him?" Describing her guest was displaying her concerns of how this man might be "babysitting" her. In paying for dinner, she stood up as powerful and obtained a narcissistic gain, although most of the time she does not feel like that.

Self-related emotions, such as pride, embarrassment, or shame, start to manifest in early childhood. Goffman (1963) used the term *stigma* for deeply discrediting attributes. He believed there is more preponderance given to the relationship, than to the attribute. Scambler (2018) classified stigma into (a) felt stigma – the individual's belief that they are likely to have a negative reaction from others because of their socially undesirable attribute – and (b) enacted stigma, when the rejection turns explicit or a person finds themself isolated as the result of their difference.

Most studies on shame address the cognitive-behavioral coping strategies of appearance (e.g., avoidance and concealment). Newell and Marks suggested that people with body image issues deal with difficulties similar to those suffering from social phobia (as cited in Bessell & Moss, 2007). Kent and Keahone (2001) and Kent and Thompson (2002) related appearance anxiety to perceived stigma caused by social norms. Individuals that engage in avoidance behavior commonly base their interpretations on unhealthy cognitive schemas. Exposure to a triggering event (e.g., a question or comment) increases appearance anxiety. The individual increasingly restricts their range of activities. Innocuous situations are found threatening and need to be avoided. In the short term, a person engages in coping strategies that ultimately serve to reinforce appearance anxiety (Rumsey, Clarke, White, Wyn-Williams, & Garlick, 2004).

Redefining the struggle of the fittest

I have been exploring the three elements that make the definition of selfhood by Cooley (1902/1922): Appearance, judgment, and feeling of mortification. Cooley is in line with Freud's (1914/1953) understanding of the body as being foundational to the ego. In Freud's own words, the ego is "first and foremost a body-ego; it is not merely the surface of an entity but it is itself the projection of a surface" (p. 3960). So, what do we project when we wish to meet others, yet remain concern about the outcome? As a projection, the judgments we come across can very well be the result of our self-beliefs and social expectations. We make the Other part of this equation.

For the drive theory, the ego is a mental representation of the individual's libidinized relationship of their body, by exposure and adaptation to reality. Our self-representation is primarily a body representation, deriving from proprioception and the experiences of pain and pleasure. Hands are the very first tools of the oral body ego (Almansi, as cited in Kestenberg et al., 1971). Hands are for learning and grasping. Later, a child will learn there are things that can be touched and other things are untouchable.

Visual communication has a significant value, to the point of being considered foundational to the ego for Lacan's (1975/2009b) mirror stage. But most of the time, we don't see with our eyes.[4] What we see finds support in primitive relationships and significant vicissitudes of our life, as well as from desire and from our efforts to be desirable. We are always playing a game of showing ourselves and seeking to be seen. At one point or another, everyone wants to be accepted and loved. We are constantly trying to make coherent the fragmented sense of who we are by searching for meaning and belonging. It is a narcissistic attempt at power and survival.

First attachments inscribe a pattern. These experiences are never forgotten. They are the early idealizations anyone can have. Subsequently, such devotion will be transferred to apropos signifiers. Beauty stands as a guiding maxima stimulus. It has also been used as a measure for classification. Thus, the ugly become outcasted. Goffman (1963) used the word *stigma* to express how an attribute could result in rejection. His conceptualization gives preponderance to the relationship, more than to the attribute that produces animosity. It is exactly this point that drives my interest.

Cooley (1902/1922) suggested that judgments can raise appearance anxiety to perceived stigma. Anxiety is a sign of helplessness, which prompts defense mechanisms such as avoidance or concealment. Furthermore, individuals who engage in avoidant behavior often determine their interpretations and according actions on unhealthy cognitive schemas. Avoidance behavior is a way of self-shunting. In rejection, we act out the demands of the representations we make based on social taste values. The ostracized have no social bond to offer shelter.

This book talks about body-related praise and criticism. In the *Origin of Species*, Darwin (2018) introduced his theory of evolution as a struggle of the fittest, in reference to strength. Each social group has a set of codes that determine what is required to fit in – beauty, intellect, strength, wealth. As a young girl, Mrs. Alem wished to be invited to the parties held at the big house. As a professor's daughter, she was invited. Yet, she felt she was "visiting," not a part of it. Even after becoming a wealthy person and moving into an expensive gated community, she continued to feel like an outsider.

Reality testing is based on an array of ego capacities and functions such as memory, mobility, attention, search, or scanning of the outer world. In this exploratory work the ego also utilizes defense mechanisms. Reality can never be perceived in the raw. A person perceives something. Nevertheless, their psychological structure, defensive mechanisms at play, primitive impressions, longing appetites, and social influences turns what is on view into an internal representation that may not be realistic. The way we perceive our body does not escape this process.

The question is whether beauty is an attribute of the thing that compels a certain emotional reaction as conceptualized by Kant (1790/2012). At risk of being found relativist, aesthetic ideas have been transformed through time and space. Therefore, it is my belief that the most genuine gesture in the judgments of taste are the feelings conceived by the judge. Such is the feeling of mortification of not finding oneself up to par with an o/Other. That is, we use people as our personal looking glasses. At the same time as we gain self-consciousness, we also idealize others, turning them into big Others. As a big Other, this person stands to represent the sociocultural realm in place.

It is my understanding that our imaginary projected judgments are an attempt to protect us from being found at fault. Participants already felt having a bodily negative attribute. In their narratives, much of what they did or did not do was in relation to how their part of the body made them feel. Mr. Horowitz said his nose "had to be kicked" more than 20 times. That "had to" shows the works of a demanding superego.

Most of participants could not tell who judged them. That did not matter. What mattered was that the weight of the ruling fell upon the body part. Even when others might not humiliate us in real life, we might still feel ashamed. In our mind they have embodied our humiliating early superego. That body part stands as the signifier of our lack.

Feeling ashamed, we keep a safe distance. We might think that by doing so, we save ourselves from the despicable things people may say about us. Unfortunately, we can hear their every word in our self-talk.

In avoidance, we do what others might do to us. In doing so, we protect them from our faults. It is a way of safekeeping the object and preserving ourselves, even when it means remaining at a distance.

Notes

1 The advantage of group action is clearly seen in a flight of birds, when they rotate to take the front place, which is more tiresome. It can be observed in the way animals assist each other at the time of laying down to sleep: Back-to-back or side-by-side in unihemispheric animals.
2 This is in line with de Saussure's conceptualization of the vertical paradigmatic relationship of the sign.
3 See Lacan (1978) Möbius strip for an example.
4 "It is only with the heart that one can see rightly; what is essential is invisible to the eye" (Saint-Exupéry, 2015, p. 24).

5 Cracked mirror, branded by shame

Shame, when our mirror cracks

Cracked Mirror, Branded by Shame is the title of my dissertation. When defending my thesis, a professor in the audience asked me why the mirror was cracked instead of broken. I was prepared for this question. Defending a thesis is a transformative occasion. It is not only about being an expert in the field, but mostly about displaying a new persona one is embracing for the first time. But that persona is not just me, it is me-within-the-audience. I want to impress them, to be accepted into the world of academia.

Once again in this book, I'll express the importance of the difference between cracked and broken. A broken mirror is one that fails to function in its reflective capacity, but a mirror that is cracked still works, although the reflection makes us feel unwholesome or questionable. Something happened in that mirroring that makes us feel ashamed. The cracked mirror is the mirror used by nonpsychotic people, the "normal" person. Those Freud called neurotics.

People use visibility as one of the means of performing and presenting identities. Mrs. Hughes, Mrs. Alem, and Mr. Alem all mentioned comparing themselves against ideals offered by the media in magazines, on TV, and so on. Comparing themselves to their neighbors or people they knew was more gentle. Whether for looks, lifestyle, or when in search of gaze, negative attributes tend to have an intensity that positive attributes fail to offer.

Shame is that feeling that comes from an uncanny discovery we make about ourselves through (real or imagined) body judgments. Many people live quietly terrified that others may think they are fat, clumsy, stinky, stupid: Inadequate. Participants talk about parts of their body. Indeed, the assumption that most everyone criticizes us is quite common. Those judgments can affect our sense of self and body image. Forty years ago, Mrs. Teak was at the front of her classroom writing on the board. One of her second grade students mentioned that she had old-looking hands. That assertion has been echoing in her mind ever since. "Not sure what that means for the rest of me," she said. Later on, she added, "As I age, my hands have aged along with me."

Judgments had a major impact on all participants, making them more "self-conscious." Most participants felt judged during their adolescence, and that incident has stayed with them ever since. During the sensitive adolescent years, outside forces become particularly important as one tries to fit into society. Self-related emotions, such as pride, embarrassment, or shame start to manifest in early to middle childhood, and they frequently relate to physical appearance. In addition, during the adolescent years an identity settles as a narrative that integrates conflicting elements into a configuration of "self-in-adult-world" (McAdams, 2001). Through the judgment they were subjected to in their life-time, participants were called upon to observe their own (real or imagined) disfigurement, which resulted in experiencing loss of integration and unity.

Touch is an early way of contact and learning. Touching is a way of welcoming shaking hands. Touch is for grabbing and keeping, as a mother holding her baby. Or its contrary, the untouchable, to eject and reject, a traumatic experience that can find their fixation point in the anal stage. Evolutionary time in which the child starts venturing themself into the world with the risk of ending up lost like Hansel and Gretel.

Erect position is also established during the anal stage. It entails mastering the vertical extension of the body, which increases the risk of falling due to gravitational force. Standing erect and tall gives a certain sense of pride. As the youngest in her family, Dr. Kamala was the baby queen. As she grew up, her brightness and queenship dwindled and faded away. She could not do long jumps. She was more of a handicapped person in needed of a stool. She associates height with recognition, respect, being accepted, and with cultural practices such as the possibility of a suitable marriage. But she is of "below average" height and feels as an "ordinary student."

Dr. Kamala was trying to improve her talents to feel bright. Her exhibitionistic wish involves showing how smart she can be and how beautifully she can recite. This wish operates in the service of self-preservation to compensate for any criticism driven by her drawbacks. She is not tall, lean, and beautiful as her ideal, and the result is an underlying feeling of inadequacy.

Like Shylock, Shakespeare's *Merchant of Venice*, Dr. Kamala's narrative is about the search for love and recognition. Dr. Kamala's mother was a bright academic. When her mother was diagnosed with schizophrenia, Dr. Kamala took refuge in the safety of her imagination and her studies. Unfortunately for Dr. Kamala, her English teacher, a nun, was her Shylock: "I was upset. Why she's doing that to me?" Her grades were low. Confused, she felt like this nun was squeezing her heart dry. Although she used to consider studying a safe space, this nun turned that safe haven upside down.

Something happens that turns our attention to ourselves in such a way that we are not simply there, but we see ourselves there, and in seeing ourselves our shame is aroused. It opens up a new level of consciousness of the self. The undivided self in action gives way to the doubled self. Shame is an act of self-attention. To know oneself is painful. In shame, we perceive the self as lacking (Schneider, 1992).

Then, one day, Dr. Kamala was asked to recite a piece from *The Merchant of Venice*: "I looked up (at the nun) and I could feel the change in her face that it was there. It means somehow her eyes were there, they developed a respect for me in her eyes because I delivered the speech so well . . ." Excelling in her recitation left her standing tall:

> I know in my heart that it was a turning point. They realized that I was very good at elocution. So they listened and I could see the change in their faces and their attitudes after they finished listening to me. And they said: "Oh! You are good. We should help you."

After that speech, the nun's "entire attitude changed." She referred to the nun having changed towards her. It is more likely that both the nun and Dr. Kamala had a transformation in attitude. Her grades changed for the better. Praise, as gaze, can be highly beneficial when considered to be sincere. It can encourage higher performance as it did with Dr. Kamala's grades.

Language has two functions – of Ereignis or coming-into-view and of sacrifice. In both, the Other is part of the equation, but one is object-related while in the latter the sacrificial object – as presented by the participants – was part of the body. As in Ereignis, which is a discrete quality, the identity of an individual also has a discrete quality that follows the natural practice of an ethos (e.g., dressing, language, behavior). In being, the individual learns, embodies social norms, and engages in proper behavior to fit in and be desirable, or decides to break out and identify themself as a rebel. The individual is vulnerable to criticism and craves fitting in.

Affective logic comes from the sensorial experiences of early times. It is preverbal, fused, and fusing. It supersedes by belonging as a way of being in the world. It is not discrete as the logic that fosters individual identity. Belonging means belonging to a kind of cultural capital that both supports and sustains someone's social significance. In belonging, the person longs for that earlier oceanic feeling attained through social network, longs for a connection that replaces what was previously experienced through the dyad, which is the first containment. Thus, shame is self related. It is a narcissistic feeling that alerts us about our self-integrity in relation to the containment, whereas guilt is the foreboding of inner condemnation (Wurmser, 1997, p. 17).

Shame and guilt can be two faces of the same coin. For instance, when shame represents the masochistic sexualized drive of guilt-driven self-punishment. Shame is an alarm that signs the risk our weaknesses being exposed earning the contempt of others. Shame is to gaze what guilt is to the superego.

Shame and guilt are intricately close emotions. Guilt is object related, whereas shame is body related. Both refer to narcissistic feelings of self-integrity. Shame is in line with the maternal care experienced. Therefore, it is developmentally earlier, funded in the partial drives of the body and pretending to taste values. Guilt is representative of the superego of the anal stage and based on moral values associated with the persona, thus, associated with the achievement of full object. It questions what we have done. Lacan (1975/2009b) said that once the child incorporates an image called I, the question set forward by the child in relation to the ideals the child lives up to is *Che vuoi? What do you want?* . . . or as I would say, *Who am I for you? I want to be your desire. But I am too scare to lose you – too scared to like you and not being liked back.*

Being is being someone for another. It is taking on a social role, as with Zelig – he was a psychiatrist at the hospital. His environment gave support to the role he took. The character taken each time was a negotiation between the realities of his inner needs and the outer demands. That is what having a persona means. I will be exploring this topic further in the next chapter.

Dr. Dillon described it in these words:

> I think there is something. . . . It's a very subtle but very powerful, . . . a cultural drive to certain praises and negativity. I don't think that the American people are willing to accept men who are overweight. All presidents are well-toned, extremely athletic. I mean Barack Obama, George Bush. . . . I mean, they are very, very athletic, and you can tell.

Scandalous remarks followed Mr. Trumps' annual physicals as people thought he misrepresented his weight. As reported in a *New York Times* article with the title, "At 243 Pounds, Trump Tips the Scale Into Obesity": "At 6 feet 3 inches tall, Mr. Trump now has a body mass index of 30.4. Anything over 30 is considered obese" (Karni & Altman, 2019).

Every culture has its ideal parameters. Wurmser (1997) presented a case in which a homosexual patient who had achieved more education than his father felt intimidated by him. "I'm not competing, look, I'm a suffering, submissive, innocent boy. I'm not a threat to anyone." By reaction formation, his patient sees himself as weak and suffering, which are painful feelings of mortification. I called them taste values because the significance of those attributes are culturally and group determined. Every culture has traits or aspects of the self to pursue and idealize, as much as those considered discrediting. As aesthetic, taste values trend between pleasure-unpleasure opposites. "Either Jacob competes, wins, and feels guilty, or he retreats, shows himself as weak, and feels ashamed" (Wurmser, 1997, p. 22). Shame here is masochistic sexualized self-aggression demanded by the need of punishment by guilt of the superego.

A judgment can be hurtful. It results in momentary ego impoverishment, thus the inability of participants to disqualify the messenger. Mrs. Hughes, who suffered from eczema during her childhood years, said, "Sometimes we can be our worst enemies. Negative thoughts are very easy to come into your mind." These thoughts make it hard to disqualify the messenger because we know they speak the hidden truth of our primary insufficiency.

What comes from the relation between the judge and the subject is horrifying and shameful. From the moment the judgment took place, Mrs. Teak stopped being a teacher. She was taken prey by the criticism for which she was targeted. Mr. Horowitz felt people did not see him but only his nose. Mr. Galeno still feels untouchable. The horror brought by the judgmental message left participants disorganized, fragmented, unable to reply to or dispute the statement. Every judgment has a drive and a cognitive element. That cognitive element can be ascribed to moral values and behaviors that aim toward an ideal body image. We question who we are and what we are for others. The cognitive element could also itself be ascribed to aesthetic emotional taste values that question what we are and what others want from us. Piaget (1979b) suggested that we learn and accommodate with every challenge imposed by our surroundings to take part in it.

There are two sources of guilt feeling. One is fear of authority figures and the other fear of the superego as the internalization of the parental authority. Out of the consternation of ending up disaffected, the ego submits itself to the demands of the guilt. For Freud, the superego is the keeper of social moral order. Klein (1931/1990) understood that guilt not only emerged from the Oedipus conflict but also from superego as representative of the father. She believed the superego appeared during the first six months of life. She also conceptualized guilt as an agent of the superego influenced from the early nourishments given by mother. Klein rarely makes any mention of shame.

Guilt as emotional pain refers to actions performed in real or imagined ways and to what is right or not. It is essentially auditory and exhorts confession (Akhtar, 2009). We worry about what we have done or how we have hurt someone. It is felt after crossing a boundary of who we "must be" imposed by the superego. In guilt, the judge is the I and is more common among individuals with obsessive-compulsive personality. Since the superego is in touch with both the id and the I, guilt can relate to action, omissions, and thoughts.

As guardians of social order, guilt feelings limit our strong and aggressive tendencies. These feelings restrain us for the benefit of the group and to keep our imaginary sense of integrity and honor intact. Restricted, they find their satisfaction elsewhere, sometimes as self-punishment, which implies a more developed structure, use of abstract symbolic thought, processes of logic rationalization, and categorical relationships. All hate and anger are aimed at fighting, avenging, mutilating. They are active. Guilt requires an act of compensation to repair the damage, to be forgiven.

Guilt raises questions of who we are as a person and what we have done. It refers to achieving and maintaining high self-esteem and a sense of entitlement, honor, and pride, emotions powerful enough to help us keep a sense of ego integrity. "It is before the Other that I am guilty. I am guilty first when beneath the Other's look I experience my alienation and my nakedness as a fall from grace which I must assume" (Sartre, 1943/1984, p. xxxii) (Figure 5.1).

On the contrary, in shame, our imperfections make us limited and expendable. We see ourselves as defective, weak, dirty, or having no control. This view utilizes visual and auditory drives that make up the gaze as developmentally prior to the superego. We are worried about what we are, how we look, and what others may say about us. There is a centrality of the body-self, and we tend to behave passively by avoiding people. In doing so, we protect the object from our shortcomings. We keep it pure and clean from our imperfections. Avoidant behavior is an attempt at keeping the integrity of the object.

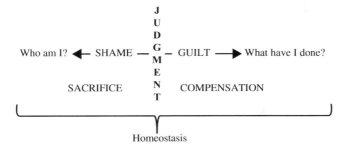

Figure 5.1 As with Mrs. Teak, in shame we question whether we are the broken pieces that our castration transpired. It requires an act of sacrifice for cleansing.

Moreover, when we question who we are and tend to feel inadequate. When we are concerned about people judging us, we hide away. We do not feel competent. We do not want to go to a party or a meeting. We can even refrain from something as simple as eating out. Avoidance is a safe place. It is both a sacrifice to preserve the purity of the object and for self-preservation. It is not an attempt to save the object itself, but for the relationship that remains as a promise. Freud believed the drive finds satisfaction on the external object or its hallucination. The drive can also find satisfaction through the path towards the object. That path is the link of our belongingness. If we consider avoidant behavior as a regressive maneuver successful at preserving both the self and the object, we can then understand how clever this artifice is. For the relationship continues at the imaginary level, as we have done so many times throughout life.

Of course, while feeling shame, we don't want to be seen. Hiding is one of the earliest defensive behaviors that comes from closing our eyes and magically believing that (whatever it is) does not exist. Staying within our comfort zone goes back to infancy, when searching for the maternal dyadic zone in which we felt safe and strong. The womb and the dyadic relationship are the archaic prototype of our sense of belonging.

Shame is earlier than guilt in the developmental line and utilizes affective logic, as well as magical thinking associated with autonomy, early narcissism, the vulnerability of the body, and the ideal self. Shame is a defense mechanism against an archaic form of vulnerability as leaving the dyad is synonym of death. There is misgiving about the loss of love, disaffection, or blunt ostracism, which can leave us as outsiders in our conquer of individualism. Mr. Whyte felt constantly judged and unwelcomed. He used eyeglasses and headphones to stop the criticism he felt coming from others. It took him some time to understand it was his own projection of an early fixation at the mirror developmental stage.

Mrs. Alem says her mother had an ideal look for her. The word *look* appears on 36 occasions in Mrs. Alem's speech. In Sartre's (1943/1984) theory of gaze, a person become aware of their own existence through others. Our feeling of shame or pride reveals us a gaze coming from others. Shame is predominantly visual. Sartre said shame is shame of oneself. Mrs. Alem tried to get closer to the ideal she held of people from the "big house." She would work hard to look just like them as a way of becoming one with them. Then, a feeling of frustration would arise, marking her distance from the ideal. At the big house, she felt like she was "visiting," not a member. She felt disgraceful when comparing herself to images from a fashion magazine. By comparing herself to average people from the streets, she felt plain and ordinary, which was better than being aware of her blemishes.

The root of the word *shame* is *skamm*, in English "wound" (Skeats, 1910). It is associated with disgrace, which historically individuals were shunned for. Shame alarms against the loss of love, of losing refuge against the odds. Participants presented fear of rejection, of not being fitted to fit in. It is not only the concern with coming across a cold shoulder what bothered the participants.

Shame alerts us of the loss of belonging, which inherits the power of our dyadic narcissistic relationships. Originally, there is an oceanic experience in the womb. Then, mother comes to maintain the illusion of that experience through appropriate actions. In children, separation from primary caregivers is equivalent to the loss of that sublime universe. It is death. Shame is awe of something sacred. In shame, we lose agency and tend toward passivity. The aggression aimed originally towards the object is turned around and inward. The drive turns onto the self and requires an act of atonement to restore and attune the conditions. Participants presented alienation of part of the self, as Mrs. Teak that was growing older and had hopes to one day be one with her hands. Dr. Dillon stated that those who are not like him are "dangerous." They are dangerous to his sense of self and belonging. They fail to support his image and make evident the distance he holds from his ideal.

As they saw their own reflection in other people's eyes through a judgment that cracked their mirror, participants felt somehow devalued, unfitting, and disfigured. Whatever happened to their body part, it resulted in a defective sense of self and an ambivalent sense of belonging. The relationship of the individual to their self and their environment ended up disrupted. The organizing or integrative function of the ego handles countless elements and systems to negotiate and achieve some level of pleasure. We all yearn for a feeling of wholeness; we covet belonging and the ability to connect with others. A part of us would rather go through life doing just about anything that allows us to reach for even a beam of that warm ray of light that we believe will enfold us when we actually get to fit properly with others.

In shame, the judge is through a gaze that comes from outside even when the judgment is imaginary. It refers to self-representation as body experience and is common among individuals with avoidant personality style and social anxiety disorder. It is developmentally earlier than guilt. Shame evolves within an economy of sacrifice to achieve atonement. Participants presented a part of their body as alienated. As dismembered, their bodies are a theater for a shunting scheme to preserve self and object. The avoidant behavior is an unconscious hide away for the preservation of those we wish to be with. Mrs. Hoocker married the only man that would not care to see her bust. He joined her in the imaginary sacrificial act that purified her sense of self. With him, Mrs. Hoocker was able to repress the highly sexual connotation of her breast and change her last name, keeping thereon a clean and proper body.

Mother is our first language. Those aesthetic values ultimately refer to safety, love, and belonging. Felt judgments are based on aesthetic taste values. At one time we were all attached to our mother by the umbilical cord. Only later do we become separate entities. We are individualized and socialized with great hesitancy. Even the illusion of stability and continuity can offer a hiding peaceful refuge to the less scared and troubled of people.

Mr. Horowitz and Mrs. Hoocker presented with self-alienation before their corrective surgery. Mrs. Teak expressed a sense of being alienated from her hand. Sacrifice is then a somatic effort for the restoration of the self (ego integration) and their ties with social reality (object relation).

Kristeva (1982) reminded us that the abject is to the superego what the object is to the ego. The abject stands at the frontier inside-outside. The superego is the guardian of our culture. Beyond that, abjection is death in symbolic terms. Identification is both, to be like the object – to hold attributes from the idealized object – and to be alienated from it. In alienation, we become an other: I'm not the person I have identified with. Only being disallowed, alienated, only symbolic death gives birth to my individuality.

Richard Schacht (2017) depicted alienation as two-fold separation: Separation from self or a part of self and separation from the true nature of the individual. This sense of estrangement implies separation and surrender. Most participants found that the part of their body they were talking about was somehow strange to them and threatening to their sense of self. Participants expressed alienation from their body part, and much of their attention was driven to this part of their body. Such alienation was an effort for integration and to secure the social bond. Alienated, this part of the body had central gravity in their lives and sense of identity. "Very often real or imagined physical attributes, parts of the body image or the entire body image, become focal points of identity" (Schachtel, 1961, p. 122). Defensive mechanisms take much of our energy.

Participants who presented a narrative centralized on one body part (e.g., Mrs. Teak's hand) spent much time and energy on the body part that they decided to talk about. They all followed their own protocol around their favored body part, as if they were preparing a mask behind which to meet the Other. Mr. Galeno – who suffered from psoriasis and craved being touched – cleaned up after himself to prevent people from having contact with his left-behind skin. Negative attributes are like eating the apple and falling out of Paradise.

6 Does it happen everywhere the same?

Puritans, old acts never forgotten

The natives had a system of knowledge based on magic (Gonzalez Taboas, 2017). In magic, truth is an emotional experience. As polytheistic, they believed in a multitude of spirits who permeated the universe as well as persons, places, and objects. Faith moves religion. In religion, there is "one God, creator of the world, legislator of the moral order" (Durkheim, 2001, p. 213). In religion, like in science, there is only one truth, which is that given by God (or validated by research).

Reardon (2012) described how Puritans' "fraternal power" helped them "achieve the solidarity and social stability to maintain their patriarchal rule over their dependents" (p. 11). The Puritans started with the idea that we are all equal under God's eyes. First, one must be God's people. Those who are not become threatening to the Puritan identity. The judgment participants received left them feeling like a freak, a stain, a sin that needs to be washed away. They feared rejection and being excommunicated. They feared becoming that abject strange other, foreigner, slave, or powerless.

Mary represents the first womb, where we flourish with an increased sense of being and belonging. As a foreclosed representation, it leaves the individual as increasingly atomistic. All the participants expressed having a disqualifying attribute that made them feel nonessential and dismissible. Becoming bizarre, different, they felt as though they had something "disgusting" or polluting, something others would not want to get in touch with, thus the understanding of this body part as a phobic attribute, as well as the lost sense of agency felt as they fell into being disposable nonentities.

In Asia Minor, Egypt, Greece, and Rome, ancient local goddess cults became absorbed into the cult of Mary (Haarmann, 1998). Orthodox Christianity calls her Panaghia. In Islam, she is called Maryam, Qānitah, or Tahira. Mary is the only woman mentioned by name in the Qur'an, and Islam pays Mary its highest compliment. For Anglicans, and many other world religions, Marian devotion exists or they have spiritual traits that can be identified as Marian (George-Tvrtkovic, 2017; Haarmann, 1998). Of course, the Jews are not devoted to Mary. Yet Judaism is a matriarchal religion. Vuola (2019) pointed out the significant absence of Mariology among Puritans in theology, liturgy, prayer, and spirituality.

In Christian theology, Mary accepted her role as Jesus' mother (Vuola, 2019). As a loving mother, she continues to intercede for all the pleas of mercy that we ask. Love is the force that helps us endure the most difficult of tasks, as in the prayers to Mary of the Sacred Heart and the Salve Regina. Love is the restorative force against fear of rejection that people carrying negative attributes as the broken pieces of themselves, of humanity, may bear. A part of their body carries heavy weight on their sense of self and finds no redemption from others when the maternal function is foreclosed.

Her imago regulates the sadism of the superego. Without her, love and life are not secured, not strong enough to counterbalance judgmental outbreaks. The participants underwent real or imagined sadistic attacks within a culture that has foreclosed the Virgin Mary's regulating function. Such events are not only attacks on the object but mainly on links. The participants felt untouchable, avoided, isolated. They felt dismembered from society. The Virgin Mary has a restorative power, but the Pilgrims did not bring her to North America. Mr. Galeno still feels no one wants to touch him, and he cleans up after himself to prevent anyone from coming into contact with his polluting skin.

The participants expressed gaining self-consciousness. Sadistic attacks transformed them into bizarre beings. They felt like freaks. The felt judgment anchored in a body part. They used protective procedures, such as covering their body with clothing to deny that body part and its message, wearing or not wearing rings as a means of controlling the message, its pith of disaffection, and relationships with others. Participants showed that the self finds its foundation in the body, initiating the question of whether they *have* or they *are* the bizarre attribute their body part represents. Mrs. Teak questioned whether she had old-looking hands or if she was old looking.

Participants embellished their body part to both attract and cover, to sacrificially alienate the bad body part and to regain good gestalt.[1] As Puritans did with the natives at their arrival, we do with the evil parts of our body. It is an attempt to control the meaning of the judgment received and the relationship with others.

For instance, in phobia, the idea is divorced from the corresponding affect of the intrapsychic conflict. The idea disappears from consciousness only to reappear in the form of anxiety linked to another idea. The phobic mind attacks (or displaces) the link to avoid contamination. Thought then remains in certitude, pure and enjoying the mental tranquility that comes from living within the homogeneous. Once purification of the body is achieved, one can only enter in association with peers.

Unfortunately, silence obstructs the mourning process of the early atrocities. They become old acts never forgotten when remaining active through unconscious processes. We have seen the collective guilt of Germans and Japanese for their offenses. Surprisingly, neither country is strong on Marian devotion. I believe the atrocities that happened in the history of the United States remain as a phobic signifier.

In phobia, the idea disappears from consciousness only to reappear in the form of anxiety linked to another idea that is innocent or worthy. Whites carry the weight of the early genocide perpetrated in the history of this country. As a phobic signifier, the repressed returns as symptomatic of all that is inequality and prejudice, becoming the driving fervor of feminism, anti-racism, or social justice of any kind. Discrimination in the form of anticipated repudiation powers the most thrusting political discussions nowadays. Popular proclamations are the symptoms of the social malaise. The risk is ending united under an ideal that gives a false sense of belonging. What makes it false? Dr. Dillon described how he aligned himself with his enemy, joining the bully group to feel protected from their judgments because of his limping. It shows that someone practicing autonomy is at risk of ending up as prey of the same group; when the glutinous effect of a shared truth gives direction and purpose and creates a moral void; where there is constraint of thought and creativity for the benefit of group indoctrination. If speech becomes a weapon, there is no room for dialogue, and freedom is given up for the good of the cause, then group alliance is not powered by the maternal function but by a sadistic superego, not by Eros but by Thanatos.

Puritans are no longer among us. Nevertheless, their influence is embedded in the American culture. My mother was a devoted Catholic. At Sunday Mass, we noticed that praying in the United States is not the same as in Argentina. In South America, we bow only once, and parishioners receive the Eucharist without lining up by rows, which allows an easier opt out. Almost every year, the feet-washing homily is about humility. The last feet-washing celebration I went to was in Missouri. To my surprise, I did not hear a word about Jesus' humble act. The homily was about service.

At the beginning of liturgy, parishioners were invited to follow the Mass using a booklet printed specially for the Holy Week. The booklet ended with an invitation to a devotional prayer after the ceremony. As an invitation, I thought it was only for those who wanted to stay. Before the priest left Mass, the whole congregation went down to genuflect for a fourth time. The choir continued singing and no one moved. At the zenith of individualism, people were behaving in tandem.

The priest came back into the chamber and sat down by the left end of the church. The choir seemed to keep on repeating the same song on and on. No one dared to move, except for one parishioner or another peeking up to check if they should remain crestfallen with hands in prayer. No one broke formation for over 20 minutes until the light went off. Only something external to the system brought the formation to an end. No one would risk being different, but my Jewish husband, who wanted to leave, patiently waited for me while asserting his ground: "Jewish people don't bow."

What bone structure can take such a strain? What God would want us to kneel for 20 minutes? It is not God but our own persecutory anxiety. We engage in behaviors that are not only for fear of discrediting attitudes, but mostly to secure our notion of comfort and stability within a world in ascending uncertainty. In a world that is exaltingly less binary, us vs. them is alive and active.

I dare say it is not them. It is us. We practice and circulate these messages. We are critical of others as part of our projections. On occasions, we celebrate the brave act of someone standing up sound and provocative against something. Freedom is not confrontation. Freedom is practicing self-honesty. If we acknowledge that on occasions we are just like Dr. Dillon, then we could also recognize that we have the power to stop the circulation of sadistic provocative practices.

Once the dyad is left behind, the true object of desire, the holding gaze that our mother offered, our experience of wholeness within the dyad, all that can never be achieved again. We can only aspire, and such aspiration needs to embrace the Other within. It is an exercise that needs to be respectful of the abject, the different, the freak, all that is not us but complements our being. To recognize the difference and embrace it is the most arduous and honest act. It does not require big acts of bravery. It really takes small gestures of kindness. Small is beautiful.

The function of the Virgin Mary and the sadistic superego

In the last three years, I have discussed the effects of judgments on people. My interlocutors and I are struck by the profound impact of body judgments presented by the participants of my research performed in St. Louis, Missouri. Indeed, everyone has a story to tell, whether they want to share it or not. It is interesting that, except for Dr. Dillon, foreign-born participants talked about more than one part of their body. For instance, Mrs. Alem presented three different body images, which she named *the tomboy,* *the nicely dressed girl,* and *the athletic woman.* Dr. Kamala talked about her height, her dry skin, legs, and other parts of her body. I called these decentralized narratives; the rest of the participants' narratives were centralized upon a particular body part: Mrs. Bryer's beautiful eyes, Mr. Horowitz's nose, or Mr. Alem's snaggletooth. That part of their body had a gravitational weight in their narrative and sense of self.

The participants' feeling of shame and anticipated rejection has a particular quality that I will try to bring to light exploring the history of colonization of North America. In an attempt to mobilize discourse, I use the term "Puritan" to distinguish the religious changes that followed the 16th-century Reformation. I will use it in a very loose way without identifying any specific religion. For Karen Armstrong (2000/2014), most Americans were Calvinists.

In the United States, self-assertiveness and self-determination are dominant personal merits. Both such qualities tend towards managing life free from the influence of others. They also express the value given to being "self-made." What happened in the history of the nation that produced an atomistic conceptualization of the human being that is the hallmark of American society? How does American culture influence the impact on judgment and consequent fear of rejection presented by the participants? What follows is an exploration into these questions and their possible answers. It is an intricate and sensitive topic; I hope you can bear with me to the end of my discussion. I write this not to be right, but to make it right.

Since the Renaissance and the Enlightenment, different conceptualizations of humanity emphasized the discrete character of individual creatures. Besides, the conception of the individual has been a useful accounting measurement for taxation, vaccination, and bearing responsibility before the law.

Unfortunately, individualism involves separation. Being an individual is a highly vulnerable condition, which is inscribed through experiences of frustration at the end of dyadic relationships and handled with various defense mechanisms. One of such defenses is taking in the representation found in the looking glass and asserted by someone in the role of the mother. The mother confirms that the image in the mirror is one's own and in doing so also sends a message of belonging.

A representation comprises affects and cultural values. Later on, we do not always have someone readily available to confirm our sense of being and belonging. Participants presented an intense fear of rejection associated with their appearance.

The Bible has various passages in which members of the Church are called "one body in Christ" (e.g., Romans: 12–5 KJV). Mary gave life to Jesus. A mother gives birth and sustains that life. It is the role of the mother to support the phantasy of omnipotence by amending needs, failures, or possible frustrations. The maternal imago supports our sense of cohesiveness and continuity, and our sense of being and belonging. Social groups are representative of the womb, whereas all the institutional norms and rules stand as representative of the superego in the role of the father.

As Jesus' mother, Mary cooperates in the redemption of humankind. The maternal imago of the Virgin Mary has a cohesive effect that emanates from her sensual and merciful figure. Unfortunately, the Reformation discontinued the veneration of Virgin Mary (Rubin, 2009). The Puritans silenced her (Vuola, 2019). I will return to this topic later to further explain its possible consequences. First, I need to present a succinct review of the history of citizenship.

The idea of citizenry involves the individual as a member of society. The earliest declaration of citizenry goes back to 539 B.C., made by Cyrus the Great, founder of the first Persian Empire, freeing the slaves he found in Babylon. By the way, he also gave them racial equality (Nice, 2014). The Romans and Greeks put citizenship in opposition to slavery. Only citizens were allowed to vote in political assemblies.

Alternatively, a king is ordained by God. Kings are above the law and rule over subjects, not citizens. A king's power lies in his sacred representation over his dominions. When a king is baptized, all his subjects are automatically incorporated into his religion, or persecuted and expelled (Christenson, 2013; Gregg, 2007). The parishioner Puritan was a member of a highly organized community, which was an advantage over mercantile colonies in North American's dawn (Horn, 2008; Chaplin, 2001/2003).

The Gutenberg's printing press, amid other advances, broadened cities and facilitated the spread of ideas. Many industrial and scientific advances started to stimulate individuals' autonomy in ways never thought of before. Markets were no longer limited to selling goods. In 1602, the Dutch East Indian Company opened the first stock exchange ("Dutch," 2019). Financial investments came into existence together with adventurous enterprises in the New World. All these changes, along with worldwide commerce, widened and sped up market interchange. A market is a place to exchange goods and services. It needs individual consumers to operate as a system of offer and demand.

I have so far mentioned three different ideas of the individual. One is religious, the second has to do with civic power, and the third is related to consumer purchasing power after the Industrial Revolution. These ideas of individualism involve agency and freedom, especially after the Enlightenment influences of Bacon and Locke. They imply religious choice, conforming to a party, or a capitalistic economy. Schooling and knowledge are offered to all while their distribution is administered to create and recreate a structure with boundaries as well as a social hierarchy. The stratification of knowledge reproduces the needs of corporate capitalism and party as two elements that work together. Capitalism is market behavior, and party is the politics that delineates a universe, its practices, and its frontiers. As a former attorney general from Argentina told me, "We are all equals under the law, but some are more equal than others."

Citizen and consumer are two ideas of individual agency. The atomistic individual is a self-directed and self-reliant unit. To paraphrase Sartre (1943/1984), an individual enjoys the freedom of decision within a set of options, which differ at every given sociopolitical temporal space. They differ from one universe to the next. For instance, individuals are free and can vote, whereas slaves and subjects of a monarchy cannot. In a previous chapter, I explore how Sartre's Other has agency, whereas the self becomes objectified when gaining self-consciousness through the Other. The individual is *me* as opposed to *you* as an alienizing Other. There is a debased quality in foreigners and slaves. Slaves lose their civic agency after being objectified by the market, whereas foreigners[2] are alienated by a cultural divide and many also suffer loss of social prestige. In Greece, Socrates (470–399 BCE) had the option of taking hemlock or departing to live as a foreigner. He chose hemlock.

Something peculiar happened in North America that shaped an outmost atomistic conception of individuality. Today individualism is at its zenith. It can be observed in the concerns of the participants of this research of not being fit to fit in. They struggled between having a negative attribute related to a part of their body and becoming the devaluated self their body part came to represent. Mr. Horowitz did not like his nose. He felt no one would like to be with a "disgusting" freak like him. For Mr. Horowitz the horror is being at risk of abjection by his superego. As a freak (a monster), he would be left as an outsider, out of the symbolic order. Negative attributes raised feelings of shame, awkwardness, and aversion. I bluntly described it as the feeling of being a "freak." The belief is that something is intrinsically wrong about one's own looks and one's own self – something so bad, so evil, no one would want to be with us.

By the 17th century, the Church had been long ruling its subjects by squeezing in heart and pockets every pain of their sin. Individuals as citizen parishioners were loved by God. Some parishioners were considered more loved than others, based on the generosity of their wallets (Santrac, 2017). Those who could not buy their absolution had to face the eternal misery of purgatory. The Augustinian monk Martin Luther included buying indulgences among the 95 complaints he had against the Church, giving birth to the Protestant Reformation (Gregg, 2007; Santrac, 2017). The world was dammed, but God could still save some of his sheep, the individual Puritan could still aim at salvation.

Puritanism did not relieve the burden of guilt. It just took away the administrators who were dispensing grace.[3] The Bible had already been translated (Santrac, 2017). The Guttenberg (1440) printing press made it accessible to most; reading literacy was the only obstacle. Puritans felt they could reach God's words directly. Years before, Wycliffe (1330–1384) determined the Bible was the only authority or representative of God, more than any earthly figure, including the Pope. Moreover, Bacon (1561–1626) suggested reason should be the only criteria of truth, even when one is seeking God's Veritas (Armstrong, 2000/2014).

In 1592, King James made Presbyterianism the official religion of England. Nine years later, he declared, "I will make the Puritans conform or hurry them out of the land" (as cited in Marshal, 1917/2011). People were fleeing by tandem; sometimes the Catholics, next the Puritans, then the Separatists. King James' proclamation of September 17, 1603, sent many offshore to Newfoundland and additional parts of the world, for they were a "great and imminent danger to the goodness of God Almighty."[4] Most of these removals ordered by the divine right of the king offered three options: "Holy resolution, divine execution or just expulsion"[5,6] (Martinez Cerezo, 2014, p. 155).

It is interesting how becoming a foreigner and death are equally holy actions aimed at harmonious living. Slaves and foreigners are abjected entities residing next to citizens. They are the phobic signifiers of the strange Other. They are a danger that needs controlling and a denial of participation to avoid contamination. The intense dread of rejection is the anticipated fright of the otherness we could turn into through shame. It involves a loss of self-agency. We fall, becoming alienated, foreign, in thrall, by our idealized members of society. We turn into *freaks*. Indeed, it is the otherness we become when the early containing mother is distant and we feel expelled out of the dyadic maternal relationship in our individualization process.

By 1620, an increasing number of the English people wanted a return to Catholicism, among them nobles and those from the House of Lords, making it more difficult for nonconformists to remain in England. Puritans and separatists left for France and the Netherlands, where they lived closer to the cities than they were accustomed to. They had to learn another language and adapt, intensifying their grief at losing identity. With the options of banishment or execution, they had no place in their old kingdom. They became abjected foreigners experiencing degradation. The concern for losing their identity poked as offensive to God. They moved to America (Bradford & Morison, 1651/2016; Christenson, 2013).

The King granted them charter powers in Virginia. The story tells that a storm took the Mayflower off course, and they ended up in Plymouth. It is likely that God inspired a new route to the helmsman (K. Voss, personal communication, May 11, 2019).

They came bringing with them the thirst for religious entitlement rather than religious freedom. Liberty could mean to them nothing but license; the very name was not compatible with their uncompromising adherence to the stern doctrine of God's sovereignty. For the Puritans, God chose them as the vessels of His truth to carry to the New World (James, 1904, p. x). Since 1570, there had been exploratory and fishing travels to Plymouth and other parts of the New World, but no permanent settlements (Paine, 2000).

Puritans felt driven by God to start anew and independent. Individuals are born again by holy water. The rebirth of the Puritans required the courage to cross an ocean. From then on, they were self-made under the all-powerful God. The King had no dominion over Plymouth. Whereas Canada was a crown colony, North America was built up as charter colonies, except for independent areas such as Plymouth.

Lévi-Strauss (1955/1988) indicated two possible options for treating what is different: (a) *antropoemia* (vomiting) – expelling the fearsome beings out of the social body – or (b) *antropofagia* – (devouring) or absorbing the fearsome forces as means of neutralizing them. Donegan (2002) suggested migrants at Plymouth believed themselves to "be" English in all essential ways – to be morally virtuous, possessing powers that set them apart, and they meant to maintain their "essence." In exile, they were fully aware that they could not go home again and that they no longer belonged to the monarchical body. It rendered a ritual of separation, as body becoming separate, "strictly covenanted to divine authority; bound not to place, but instead to its own image . . . o endure isolation, and to suffer affliction without dissolution" (Donegan, 2002, p. 19). The Puritans radically excluded, defaced, and enslaved all those who were different.

It is possible that being "self-made" was a positive character trait. Indeed, arriving in a land that had nothing but hard work awaiting the pioneers, being self-made could have been a sign of the good fortune of being chosen by God, a sign of being resourceful by the sagacity to overpower any unexpected event the New World could offer. As a religious community, the Puritans were more organized, free, and healthier than many other newcomers (Chaplin, 2001/2003; Horn, 2008). Their ethos spread as new colonies were created. They had the Bible as a premier object of truth with God's rationally justifiable assertions. Nobility and State social status was replaced by social class, giving privilege to the first comers and the Founding Fathers. Everybody is the same, but some are more equal than others.

The Mayflower arrived at the beginning of winter. Death and hunger were a real threat. About half of the newcomers died the first year during travel or once arrived (Chaplin, 2003). The Pilgrims would have never survived without the generosity of the natives. The relationship between the natives and the Pilgrims was amiable until the Pequot War of 1636. Plymouth condemned the territorial intrusion and harsh actions of the English people from Massachusetts. Still, in 1643, they joined Massachusetts and Connecticut in forming the New England Confederation. Over the years, relations grew aggravated. The population grew in North America, and new Europeans came to conquer the West. Military security was a method of preserving a certain way of life. The natives were isolated and moved into reservations (Russell, 2002).

Every year at Thanksgiving, we are told the early Pilgrims would have perished without the assistance of the natives. We celebrate that first mythical event as a story of origin and therefore of the creation of the United States of America. It follows a perverse logic, of admitting the importance of the natives to later feeling entitled by God's grace to free the tribes of their wildness and contain them within reservations. For the newcomers, being America's keepers was God's destiny. The mindset brought by the Pilgrims was still active two centuries later when Brigadier General Don Forrester Pratt suggested the dictum "kill the Indian to save the man" (Pratt, as cited in Russell, 2002, p. 66). It is still active today in messages like "I am a man" (1968), "Hands up don't shoot" (2014), "I am a child" (2018), and many others.

The natives were isolated on reservations, instructed not to speak their language, tearing away their offensive rituals to civilize them into society one by one.[7] The natives were considered to have an "imperfect conception" and a "savage nature," "torn to pillage" and against "the maxims of the white man's morality" (*Ex Parte Crow Dog*, 1883). The Cherokees filed a complaint with the Supreme Court. Surprisingly, the Cherokees won their case. The Supreme Court recognized them as "people capable of maintaining the relations of peace and war. They look to our Government for protection, rely upon its kindness and its power, appeal to it for relief to their wants, and address the President as their Great Father" (*Cherokee Nation v. Georgia*, 1831). Nevertheless, Cherokees and further tribes were treated as aliens and deposited on reservations. A series of forced relocations of Cherokee, Chickasaw, Choctaw, Muscogee, Seminole, and many tribes followed.

I drove through Chattanooga, a mountain area in Tennessee where the Trail of Tears passed. It was a painful zigzag in a comfortable car. I cannot imagine what it was like to walk the Trail of Tears hungry, debilitated, and not knowing what to expect. Thousands died on the way (Foreman, 1989). As the natives walked into the reservation, their names were taken one by one. It is an old tradition of membership in parishes. The natives relocated into reservations were converted into a new bureaucratic term: American Indians The only official Indian tribes are those created and certified by the Bureau of Indian Affairs, which was created in 1824 by John Calhoun, Secretary of War (Haake, 2017; Russell, 2002).

Not every native went onto a reservation. Yet, the only people allowed by law to call themselves American Indians in the United States are the descendants of those who entered a reservation and are holders of a Certificate of

Degree of Indian Blood by lineage. The removal finished with the natives and turned them into American Indians, which is a western creation and first shunting act in the history of this country. American Indians became the phobic Other of the "American Holocaust" (Stannard, 1994) or "American Genocide" (Madley, 2017). The representation of the American Indian has prevailed as a phobic signifier of what is foreign or alien.

Some natives were auspicious and acquired European fashion and costumes, thus embracing the difference with their strange Other. The idea of private property, free of any duty to render service to King and Crown, was new to the Puritans (Vance, 1924).[8] For the natives, land was sacred, lived off, a place of hope, tradition, and nurturance they identified with (Wolfley, 2016). For many Indigenous people, land is not owned but inhabited. Those who own land and have more than they can work themselves need hands to operate it. In came the Africans to work the land. Skin tone was an easy-to-spot badge used for classifying slaves and natives from Whites. Such classification gave origin to what we now call discrimination. The moment "Indians began to relate servitude to color, the seeds of racism were sown" (Russell, 2002, p. 70).

The variety of testimonies and demonstrations associated with the history of African Americans by White Americans is surprisingly vast. I have not seen mention of the slave relationship between American Indians and African Americans in a museum exhibition yet. Would this reflect the Whites' self-reproach? Shortly after my arrival as a foreign graduate student in St. Louis, I was criticized when mentioning the history of Irish indentured servitude in the United States after the terrible history of hunger and wars in Ireland. The course was on cultural diversity.

For me, skin tone differences brought nothing but good memories. I must have been around six years of age when I was walking hand-in-hand with mamá through the streets of Buenos Aires. When I asked her about it, she said something like: "God created variety to make life more interesting." As a graduate student, I was astonished. I quickly learned I was Latina and something like a chocolate croissant – brown inside with White looks. In the 1870s, Argentina executed a military campaign called the Conquest of the Desert against many natives. However, *mestizo*,[9] *mulato*,[10] and *criollo*[11] are ways of acknowledging the reality of mixing the old with the new, producing something original. My world until then had never been Black or White. There was no oreo, apple, or coconut. I only became Latina when I moved to the USA. Classifying the inhabitants of a country is in my experience, an American practice that is currently under high level of disgrace. But we cannot deny history. We have to accept it. Accepting out painful past is the healing path. It helps us change towards a better future,

In history, many events are not part of the official narrative. It happened in the United States as it does in many other places. Some facts remain under the rug, beyond the boundaries of a simplified social imaginary.[12] Having one story is like enjoying the glutinous effect of a shared truth that supports the safety of all individuals within the system. It gives direction and purpose. "The quest for total coherence and the elimination of difference and plurality lead eventually to the death of the symbolic but also to a moral void" (Wieland, 2015, p. 22). Going beyond that is like crossing the frontier with the risk of ending up ostracized as others have been before.[13]

To use Symington's (1990) terms, the God that arrived was narcissistic and self centered. "Then God said, 'Let us make man in our image'" (Genesis 1:26, KJV). The Pilgrims arriving into North America introduced patriarchy as the natural order of things. Women did not vote in Puritan assemblies, albeit the predecessor of Puritanism, John Wyclif (1330–1384), suggested in one of his sermons that it would be impossible "to obtain the reward of Heaven without the help of Mary" (as cited in Divozzo, 2019, p. 3). Puritans criticized the worship of anyone other than God (e.g., saints, martyrs, or Mary), because their adoration was but a distraction (Clark, 1969/2015; Vuola, 2019). "For there is one God, and one mediator between God and man, the man Christ Jesus" (Timothy 2:5, KJV). Puritans brought God without the mediating function of Mary's love.

For Clark (1969/2015), Puritans tend to conceive their God as male. On the contrary, Orthodox Church, Christians, and a variety of religions are deeply devotional of Mary. Thus, their God has a "feminine principle" (p. 177). The symbolism and imagery of Mary generates a different set of experiences (Driver, 2013). Her imagery is that of a powerful divine protector (Vuola, 2019).

"A boy or a girl who has a conflict with God may take a detour through the mediation of Mary's obvious maternal and compassionate intercession or resort to some saint with peculiar affinities with him or her" (Rizzuto, 2004, p. 439). As a good enough mother, the function of the Virgin Mary stimulates tolerance of frustration and encourages openness and flexibility to endure the mysteries of life. The Madonna turns doubt into a force that inspires curiosity and sagacity for adventuring into the world. Her purity and grace beams virtue into our hearts as a protective layer to all. Salve Regina instills compassion, hope, and forgiveness. The God of the Puritans brought to the New World thrust the reign of a sadistic superego without Her regulating sensual figure to compensate for our feelings of guilt and shame and to help us overcome sadistic attacks.

Spain, Portugal, and southern Italy were devoted to the Virgin Mary (Symington, 1990). Her image gained substance among polytheist Latin American natives by the blend of Christianity and Pachamama (Mother Earth) (Mariscotti, 1978).[14] Puritans colonized the United States, bringing a religion free of distracting influences. The Eucharist and Virgin Mary stayed at the shores of the southern coast of England. For the French Reformer theologian, Théodore de Bèze (1519–1605), women should have a traditional household role:

> As long as she lives,
> She must seek her husband's pleasure
> And be in perfect control of all she does
> So that she should never do anything
> Which displeases him.
>   ("The Role," n.d.)[15]

As in many native groups, the Lakota Sioux believe the Sun represents the universal Father and the universal Mother is the Earth. Thus, women had a high social standing in patriarchal Lakota tribes. Other tribes were matrifocal (Jaimes, 1982; Portman & Herring, 2001). American native women lost their status because only American Indian males could sign treaties with the United States government and European monarchies. Colonial government was based on votes from all free men[16] but no women.[17] In 1870, the United States granted the vote to Black men. It took another 50 years for women to achieve the national right to vote. Women had no national voting rights until 1920 with the 19th Amendment. Once again, in 2008, the Democratic Party had to choose between the first African American man and the first female presidential candidate. Obama, the African American, was elected. In 2016, Clinton lost again, this time to Trump. Furthermore, women have been losing their maiden last name when married, which can be interpreted as a property that passes from father to the new spouse. In Latin America, women add their spouses last name to theirs. Their children carry both parents last names.

Notes

1   The child identifies with the image in the mirror even if exposed to negative messages during childhood. Mrs. Clayton is an example of that.
2   Since the 12th century, European immigrants were common in England. Foreigners had restricted residency rights. They were not allowed to work at the market or pray at local parishes. Only by paying special taxes could they gain some rights (Bartel, 2006). Shakespeare made many references to the reputation and status of foreigners in *The Merchant of Venice* (2017), *Othello* (2015), and *Measure for Measure* (2006).
3   The Puritans considered the Bible an authority "in all matters of Christian faith and practice" (Dreisbach, 2017, p. 24), and "Jesus should simply be revered as a great teacher, the founder of a remarkable, simple, exalted, and practical religion" (Armstrong, 2000/2014, p. 73).
4   Puritans were not the only ones expelled. During the Middle Ages, England and surrounding islands suffered intermittent pandemics, famines, and wars that left many homeless and begging. Rogues, vagabonds, idle, and dissolute persons were sent to Newfound Land (American continent), the East and West Indies, France, Germany, and Spain (Brigham, 1911/2014).
5   Both in Spain and England, removals were ordered by divine right of the king (Martinez Cerezo, 2014).
6   My translation.
7   An 1824 letter from various Cherokees to Secretary of War Calhoun reads they have become "a prey, defrauded out of their lands, treated as an inferior being on account of their poverty and ignorance; they became associated with the lowest grade of society" (Haake, 2017, p. 38).
8   For Vance (1924), Plymouth enjoyed allodial tenure. Commercial charters were under common socage (Connecticut, 1821). Bethell (1998) explained how the Puritans' travel was financed by Thomas Weston, from London, with the arrangement that "everything would be divided equally between investors and colonist" at the end of seven years. Once arrived at Plymouth, working in communal property was not as easy. The industrious workers were forced to subsidize the slackers or free-riders. Eventually, Bradford decided to subdivide the plantation and gave an acre per individual, (Bethell, 1998; Bradford & Morison, 1651/2016).

9 Someone of Spanish and Indigenous descent.
10 Someone of Spanish and African descent.
11 Someone of Spanish descent and autochthonous of Latin America
12 Social imaginary, imaginario social in Spanish.
13 As an example, in October 1635, Roger Williams (1603–1683), Puritan minister and founder of Rhode Island, was banished for spreading "new and dangerous opinions." He believed in buying land from the natives, freedom of conscience, and the prohibition of slavery (LaFantasie, 1988).
14 In his song Santa Evita, Andrew Lloyd Webber observed how many Argentines pray to Evita Perón as an actualized Virgin Mary's imago.
15 This preaching appears as much a ruling for the behavior of women before their husband's as a dictate for how men behave before God. As in Hobbes (1651/2013), "I know thou wilt command thy children and thy house after thee to keep the way of the Lord" for the obedience of his family "depended on their former obligation to obey their sovereign . . . All subjects are bound to obey that for divine law" (pp. 176–177). Furthermore, preaching against "outrageous behavior" that restricts the display of aggression is noteworthy and still current in the United States, where there are limited acceptable outlets for the display of aggression.
16 "Puritans were horrified by the idea that citizens might try to use their right to vote to promote their own individual interests. The role of voters was to assist the magistrates in promoting true religion" (Lombard, 2003, p. 149). "Voting rights were only offered to church members." Brethren, or full members of the colony's Congregational churches had "absolute political and juridical authority" (Reardon, 2012, p. 74).
17 The "society founded by Puritans in early New England was based on a hierarchical world in which fathers ruled, by virtue of their ability to rationally govern a passionate, uncontrolled, and sensual majority of dependent women, youths, children, servants, and enslaved Africans. . . . The Puritans envisioned society as a "series of hierarchical relationships, in which fathers' authority within the polity and their authority within the family were homologous. The ideology of patriarchal manhood provided the foundation for one form or seventeenth-century patriarchalism" (Lombard, 2003, p. 12).

7 Being and belonging

On being

The verb to "be" can be translated into Spanish in its temporal (*ser*) and spatial (*estar*) meanings. Being in its temporal connotation is an action-based way of living. In the United States, when asked "Who are you?", people tend to answer with a name and a degree or job description.

In individualistic societies, people grow up learning to think of themselves as "I." This "I" is classified according to individual characteristics. Once children are grown, they are expected to leave their parental homes, reducing the relationships with their parents or breaking off with them. The North American individual pursuits of being assertive, self-reliant, effective, and succinct (Hofstede, Hofstede, & Minkov, 2010), result in a depravity of contact.

Hofstede et al. (2010) described the United States as a "masculine" culture. In the United States individuals suffer from anxiety[1] (Alonso et al., 2018) and loneliness[2] (Cigna, 2018). The individual trembles hesitantly at the wish of enjoying even a flare of that delight essence that comes from being with others. Cautiously, they cave in, ending up isolated in their own self-made balloon. Anyone can forge up shelter. Unfortunately, isolation tends to increase paranoid defenses. In a defensive way, they set up increasing levels of control and isolation. The individual starts by rejecting the stranger for self-preservation, when perpetuation is dependent on our relationship with others. It is a cycle. We are social beings regardless of the cherished personal traits of a given culture.

Knowledge and control are common ways of regulating highly stressful emotions. A few weeks ago, I was closing Mrs. Sawyer's case. She mentioned that she finally "felt (she) did not need to know it all" – that she "was now able to give herself time to search for an answer." Not knowing, not being able to prepare herself for any eventuality, had been highly distressing for Mrs. Sawyer.

I am not talking about a knowledge that incites understanding and wisdom. On the contrary, these qualities require awareness and curiosity and such attributes originate from the maternal function. We can see it in a toddler who adventures into the world so long as a representative of the dyadic haven is present in real or imaginary ways. Gonzalez Taboas (2017) acknowledges having seen many atheists and agnostics turn onto praying in times of need. Thus, it can be observed in the many who seek assistance from Mary during challenging moments to grasp a tad of the confidence she once had: "Be it unto me according to thy word" (Luke 1:38 KJV) or to find inspiration and courage: "If Mary can go to Heaven, I can go to Congress" (Nancy Pelosi, as cited in Singer, 2010, p. 238).

Some questions sting right where our feelings of inadequacy arise, especially for those growing up in a masculine culture in which the superego is hard to balance. Hurtful judgments poke at our primary insufficiency. The participants of this study embodied their feelings of inadequacy in a specific body part. Such practice is not new; countless times, psychoanalysts have shown the somatic participation in psychic afflictions. The way participants managed the judgments about their body was aimed at preserving their narcissistic and object cathexes.

Participants presented denial and alienation of their particular body part. A sacrificial act of purification allows them to align with the ideal and to be worthy of object relationships. Consequently, preserving the matrix of belonging.

Toddlers take parental rules as something to live by. It is part of their survival to be a desirable child. Even adults may relish the comfort and tranquility of following other people's commands. Part of being an adolescent is making relationships beyond the immediate family and deciding what parameters work for us. Winnicott (1986) used to say the adolescent needs to overthrow the king. Up until then, a child follows different lines of development. The last frontier is no longer a progressive biological maturity. This last act of maturity within the family is accepting the responsibility for actions, but mostly for our future. It is a paradigm shift, from being for our parents to being for ourselves.

To avoid the risk of being simplistic, let us admit that individualism is not limited to the United States. Nevertheless, in this country, an "extreme form of American individualism" has arisen (Campion, 2017, p. 114). Today, neighbors in cities remain strangers (Dunkelman, 2017). It is my understanding that this is at least in part a consequence of the history of this country. Personally, I consider letting teenagers leaving their family unit as a repetition of that early departure from Europe.

The Puritans arrived at Plymouth, and from then on, there was little option but to be self made, self reliant, and assertive. They left behind the structure of a city or village. They turned their backs to all that was known to them for a place that offered opportunity but had no community structure other than their own religious congregation to fall back on. Collective action offers meaning when human beings fear loss of identity or feel helpless. Citizens can exchange obedience for protection against the threats to their existence (Bauman, 2000/2018). The Puritans obeyed God's will to gain His protection.

Unfortunately, since the birth of this nation, Puritan influence has resulted in a culture that generates a deficit in structural self-object relationship building that makes individuals particularly vulnerable. For Bauman (2000/2018), people's susceptibility is due to the absence of social stability, the eroded certainties of global economies, and monadic individualist identity.

An individual grows in interaction with their environment through different developmental lines or networks with successively increasing differentiation and hierarchical integration. This process is full of cultural and emotional influences. In adolescence, there is a developmental paradigm shift. Historically, the individual changed family of origin for social groups, searching for a companion and the creation of a new family structure. Adolescence has always been a difficult and conflicted developmental stage. The participants received their judgments during this time. Their body-related judgments put at risk their sense of being and belonging. Maybe now, for those growing up in liquid environments, the adolescent is an anonymous, replaceable, atomistic individual in constant worldwide competition. Rivalry starts even before the constriction of family life is left behind in seeking one's own place in the world. There is an effort to follow utilitarian morality. Lacan (1975/2009b) called it *Che vuoi?* In the search for being, we need to be something for someone, even when we might deny it to reduce susceptibility but that search – or the susceptibility of being fit to fit in – has not changed.

Words such as *discrimination, perpetrator*, and *bullying* are far more than expressions. They explain many real things that can happen with intense apprehension. They create representations of what to look after, especially in a country where children have gone from practicing nuclear bomb drills at school to being prepared for shooting incursions. When someone is assigned an evil role, others must find refuge.

Except for Hollywood movies, American culture is highly dismissive of any explicit aggressive display. Passive aggression is far more common. Expressions such as *bullying, perpetrator*, or *discrimination* can result in tunnel vision. They offer a script of how people should behave. Mr. Appleby was 15 years of age when he felt his schoolmates were taking advantage of him. Did he feel awkward and like he did not fit in? Was he displacing something that was happening at home? The day after his birthday, he went to school and punched a chair with all his fury. He was not allowed back, thus increasingly affecting the already painful feelings of isolation and misunderstanding. In being-as-action, there is no time for listening. He says no one asked him why he did that, not even after hurting his hand. No one listened. Instead, his mother sent him to a psychiatric institution for inpatient care for two weeks. He felt sent away, and he continues to live apart in a world of his own; as he described it: "My boss let me set up my office, so it fits my needs." He relates to objects and animals more easily than to people.

Once the kings and queens are overthrown, the adolescents of the 1970s wanted to enjoy freedom and to have the responsibility of creating their own path. Years later, in the liquid society of our times, freedom involves a rebuff of attachments. There is no responsibility other than to oneself. Being autonomous means being self-normed. The individual attempts to control any potential harm. Ego-knowledge overpowers anxiety. Lacan (1969/2007) described the scientific discourse as coming from knowledge (savoir) that is imparted to another, dominating it. The hegemony of knowledge is used to control the other and masks the reality of our fragmentation.

The individual is a monad whose identity persistently needs reshaping. The body is one of the few constant objects someone can have in the liquid reality. As a consumer, the individual acknowledges being an object in the market. The utilitarian environment encompasses the manipulation of bodies happening in its virtual and real dimensions. For some, belonging is an aggregation of Internet followers. It is not so much a bonding experience of trust and support as trust and support are transient expressions of mechanical solidarity.

Ms. Ralph recently started dating after spending five years with the same boyfriend. She stated she had "friends with benefits to satisfy her sexual needs." Most of these friends are "not compatible for long-term relationship" because they "lack motivation, have children of their own, use alcohol or drugs," the list continues. Sex and love have parted ways. For Ms. Ralph, thinking of going on a one-time date shields her from the mortification of wishing for a follow-up rendezvous that does not happen. She craves the sweet-sounding mellow feeling of connection found in love or does not crave it at all to avoid frustration. Her surroundings appear to impose a tiresome journey as she reformulates and seeks what clicks on her sense of being and belonging.

Case I: Mrs. Teak

Mrs. Teak is dressed in fashionable clothes. She wears make-up and plenty of jewelry. During most of the interview, I feel excited listening to her talk. She described herself as a teacher and a mother. Oftentimes, our professions involve using and exposing the body. This is the case of Mrs. Teak, when "back in the day" she had to stand up in front of her students and write on the chalkboard. "I used to write on the chalkboard, so they'd see your hands more." Nowadays teaching is "completely different." That is how Mrs. Teak felt exposed to her students' observation of her having old-looking hands.

For Bisagni (2009), hands support speech. Hands can communicate by use of gestures, writing, making music, or discerning sensory information by the blind. Hand-eye coordination is basic for interacting with our environment. Through touch we are able to apprehend and learn in active or passive ways. Hands are used to grasp, carry, push, hold, count, weigh, and find or give pleasure. "In fact, 'hand' is really a synecdoche for 'body'" (Aragno, 2011, p. 275). The hand holds the thumb, which is the finger supporting mother's representation when she is not there. We first explore space with the use of our hands, gaining a double representation of belonging to the body as well as to the space into which we grow and reach. Hands are the primary tool of the oral body ego (Almansi, as cited in Kestenberg et al., 1971). Hands are useful for protection and connection. We "shake hands," "give a hand," "show a hand," or ponder what's "on the other hand." We can notice something "at first hand," have a "sleight of the hand," "wash our hands" as Pontius Pilate did, or end "hands up."

Ever since a pupil spoke his callous truth, Mrs. Teak has felt her hands were old looking. It opened an enigma, a psychic wound. She started by telling her students "not to say 'that'" – which she could not even mention. She tried to identify her hands' features as an inherited family trait. She used cream lotion, hid her hands, entertained the idea of using fatty injections, and checked the effect of gaining or losing weight. All these strategies helped her deal with the meaning of a message that is embodied in her hands. Her answers are mechanisms of defense such as identification, disavowal, or phantasy.

> Well, I've, ah, I would say I've been criticized with my hands. I'm very, uhm, and it's been for a long time cause now that I am getting older but I still have very old hands for my age . . .
>
> Um, when I was a teacher, sometimes kids would comment as I would write on the board, things like that, so, uhm, I try to use − I think it − I think I, I became more self-conscious of it.
>
> I've always been, you know, as a teacher, pretty honest with them and I said, 'You know, it kinda hurt my feelings and everything,' and, and they pretty much stopped.
>
> Luckily kids are brutally honest.
>
> I don't think they're coming from a malicious [place], you know.

When Mrs. Teak heard the judgment given on her hands, she started processing by evaluating the message, its source, the truth in it, and whether it was believable. For instance, "People are more critical of the way you look," whereas children don't "come from a malicious" place. Finally, Mrs. Teak considered who to believe. "Kids are brutally honest" and her friends would not be as honest because "they wouldn't want to hurt her feelings." Since the original message was provided by a kid, and "kids get to say anything they want without a filter," the message must have been somehow true as Mrs. Teak repeatedly questions its validity. She never thought about her old-looking hands before, but its significance has been echoing in her life ever since.

> So, then I . . . I became a little more self-conscious and I would look, I would notice other people's hands, noticing that they, you know, looked a lot younger.
>
> Ah, well, it made me feel bad 'cause I had never heard it before, you know? I didn't think about it before but I, looking back, I remember like my grandfather had hands like these.
>
> It's, like I said, it's, it's kind of inherited but my sister doesn't have hands like this so I think, I think I was more aware of it and of course I was 20 so I was fairly young when it happened.
>
> Uhm, well, by that time I've already been told by my classroom that I had old hands and I kinda said: You know, you're right. You're right I have, you know, older looking hands.

In the judgment of old-looking hands expressed with brutal honesty by a child, Mrs. Teak learned how society perceived her. She took the message with ambivalence. It was a judgment regarding part of her body that resonated with

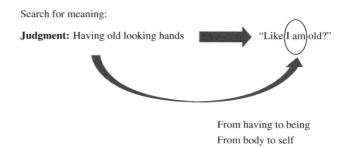

Search for meaning:

Judgment: Having old looking hands   "Like I am old?"

From having to being
From body to self

Figure 7.1 Mrs. Teaks repeats the judgment as if she were a carrier of other people's messages

the rest of her persona with an inquisitive hesitation: "Like I am old?" She is aware, acknowledges, and admits that she has old-looking hands to later reject or conceal this same element. It could be that accepting that she is old looking like her hands involves an attribute of lesser value in our society, and she rejects being old. Furthermore, old age is associated with death and Mrs. Teak was 20 years of age when she heard a kid speak his truth (Figure 7.1).

Striving to fit in, a person usually takes the character's role and benefits from recognition. Since Mrs. Teak listened to the social judgment, she conceived it as a foreign truth ("you are right") that she was willing to accept. She adapted to what she perceived others wished for her. She appears willing to admit that her hands carry the value of other people's message ("I have"). The aggression of that judgment remained embodied in her old-looking hands for 40 years with masochistic gain. The initial experience opened an enigma that Mrs. Teak spent 40 years reinterpreting, elaborating, and more than anything, defending herself.

Listening to Mrs. Teak talk, one has the impression that her hands are a part of her that is somehow apart: "As I aged, my hands have aged along with me." Almost like having a body and a fraction (her hands). The judgment contained in the message has an indeterminate effect, "Not sure then what would that mean for the rest of me . . ." The body is the foundation of the self. Mrs. Teak is troubled by a narcissistic wound. As with any narcissistic wound, it makes the whole into a part – her hands and the rest of her. Anchoring the conflict in her hands, she ends up questioning her persona, "Like I am old?" In a sacrificial act that keeps the purity of her sense of self, she remained alienated from that evil part her hands are for her. Yet at the end of the tunnel there is hope: "So now, I think I'm growing into them." This statement seems to convey an emergent element of hope in regaining a good gestalt for as she grows older her hands and her body will finally be a match, a one whole body.

On belonging

For Hofstede et al. (2010), in masculine cultures such as America, esteem prevails over belongingness. Yet participants of this study showed high concerns over not being fit to fit in. Thus, even in the most individualistic of cultures, human beings seek socialization. The verb to "be" can be translated into Spanish in its temporal (*ser*) and spatial (*estar*) meanings. The spatial connotation of being emphasizes the roots that bring about our being in the world, as well as the experience of belonging. Allowing oneself to feel a sense of connection with our surroundings does not always involve a welcoming experience, as the participants made clear.

Belonging is the ground of a figure, the negative on a painting, the sound that holds together musical notes. It is the experiential reservoir that makes possible understanding without words. Within the vibration of those elements, the essence of a glimmer brings me from the shadows. I belong in this transitional space between me and others. In belonging, we overcome the separation of our bodies to feel, once again, the chemistry of reunification.

The original sense of belonging is experienced within the dyad; thus, it follows the affective logic. It starts within that space between two bodies in symbiotic relation and from there, it spreads out with the rhythms of maturity. Belonging is an inherited creation of the leftovers of the dyad. It is represented in successive relations creating a matrix from where my sense of being in the world stands, a matrix that sustains and supports the social significance of a person.

There are endless signifiers that can be used as dimensions of belonging. Nevertheless, measuring it is taking an aspect as a totality while denying its wholeness. The attempt to gather attributes of belonging is using rational conceptualizations to access something originally cultivated by the affective logic. Identity, as belonging, is not set on stone. We are constantly reshaping our identity narratives and renegotiating those qualities that bring us closer or distant, that make of us members or outsiders, that make us feel more or less. Our identity narratives respond to our sense of self, and we create or recreate our narratives based on how we feel and how we negotiate the many elements and defensive mechanisms active during our standing in the world. But we cannot escape belongingness.

Local belonging is later associated with social, geographical, and cultural roots. It is a community practice of solidarity. Its territorial anchor acts as reference and is the source of identity and life orientation. There is a sharing of cultural symbols and meaning. In its healthy form, its boundaries are flexible with enough levels of tolerance for adaptation. The Internet has brought new ways of connecting and belonging. I am inclined to believe the maternal function of the Virgin Mary can strengthen the sense of belonging, thus making judgments less upsetting or discrediting.

"Americans are seldom exposed to ideas outside the silos of their own experience. Neighborly conversations might puncture the bubbles that otherwise develop when you talk almost exclusively either to your closest acquaintances or your similarly oriented peers" (Dunkelman, 2017, p. 55). The individualistic American culture fostered isolation and avoidance instead of connection and rapport. Bonding does happen but within a group of equals. As with Dr. Dillon, it takes place with comrades that are willing to surrender to the group for group protection. The members of the group can no longer crack our mirror for they have ascribed to the group at the expense of their freedom, for freedom may crack the mirror.

Case II: Dr. Dillon

Dr. Dillon is a fifty-something immigrant professor. He is tall, trim, and recently started to let his hair grow. At the time of the interview, his hair was curly, untidy, and reached his shoulder. He has noticed that people tend to despise this look, "But my girlfriend likes it." There is an almost undetectable limp in his walk because one of his legs is shorter than the other one. When I first asked him if he had ever been praised or criticized for the way he looked, he mentioned his limping ordeals. At the time of the interview, which lasted over an hour in a most relaxed atmosphere, he decided to share a different story.

> Mm-hmm . . . The first time I really encountered a criticism of my body was when I was with neighbor kids, cycling in the streets in Switzerland. And . . . Uh! It was a hot summer day so I took off my shirt and . . . and one of the kids turned to the other and said: "I would be ashamed if I had a fat belly like this one." And I was shocked! Truly shocked, I was not even aware that I had a belly.

His story started when he encountered an athletic second grade kid that he barely knew. As he got the message, Dr. Dillon crashed into western values embodied in the voice of a young boy: "A fat belly like this one." Although Dr. Dillon grew up in a strongly conservative family, he seems to have been shielded from certain western values until that moment of sudden awareness. "I think the kid was acting out something he heard, and I think it has to do with the culture that you have to look fit." Dr. Dillon believed that, at the time, he "had no self-defense mechanism in place" to properly respond to such a contention. He had no way to say "Oh yeah! That's complete nonsense." Because the kid spoke turning onto another youngster, it is also unclear if the message was directed at him. Such a judgment "left a major impact on me. . . . It made me a little bit more conscious. I even remember that after almost 50 years. . . . I think that's sitting somewhere in the background of my head even if I'm consciously not aware of it."

Dr. Dillon views himself as a "rebel." That is, as someone who "did not conform to the conservative views" of western society, values emphasizing "athletic, muscles, uh, young-looking, youth is appreciated. . . . So there is an appraisal and that's the role model, that's how you should look like." However "rebel" and nonconforming he might be, this experience had a lifelong impact. It could at least raise an eyebrow as he states that he does not care for the western values by which he lived most of his life. "So I think there is something. . . . It's a very subtle but very powerful, uh. . . . cultural drive to certain praises and negativity."

I . . . I don't think that the American people are willing to accept men who are overweight. All presidents are well-toned, extremely athletic. I mean Barack Obama, George Bush. . . . I mean, they are very, very athletic. They have good workouts, personal trainers, and you can tell.

Dreading being "eradicated" by his looks, he tried to distance himself from any feelings of desertion. He projected them onto the Americans, even though this incident happened back in Switzerland. It should be noted that he later chose to live in this country.

By fifth grade, "strangely enough, I was strongly built. . . . I was the fastest runner. . . . I was strongly built but . . . but there was still a limp in my run." That "but" shows his personal dissatisfaction. Although he had developed an athletic build, moving toward the western hegemonic masculine ideal, he felt unable to comply. Shame, disgrace, or disgust seemed to kick in when he found himself at a distance from the ideal. Until recently, he avoided going to the beach and places where he should be without a shirt. He shared the restlessness of having felt fingered: "Ugh, look at that belly," or "Look, I wouldn't . . . I would not dare to take off my t-shirt if I would look like him, or something." About 40 years have gone by, and the words of that child riding his bicycle still resonate in his head. Dr. Dillon craves being able to take his shirt off. There is an exhibitionist drive, followed by the kid's message echoing in him. If people were to look at him they would find him not fitted, and he very much wants to fit in. I asked, "If there were something wrong with you, what would happen? What would that mean?" He replied, "I would be not accepted. . . . As a kid, you want to be accepted in your peer group. I instinctively knew, you know, you want to be on the good side of them (the dominant group)."

Dr. Dillon showed concerns of being bullied due to his limp, and he wished to belong. He wanted to feel "integrated" and "protected." Next, he appeared to turn a negative into a positive: "The irony is I always wanted to be a little bit of a rebel. I always thought it was not maybe a kinship, but there's curiosity, people who are different, who could not, or would not, or don't want to fit in. I thought they were always interesting." Turning a negative into a positive or turning rejection anxiety into an inclination towards being a rebel is a defensive maneuver. Dr. Dillon finds some "kinship" in those who are different. His statement is the expression of a narcissistic drive. Dr. Dillon could identify himself with his Iraqi and Turkish students who feel ostracized, but he does not. He finds them impossible to connect with, maybe even weak. He sees them suffering in a role whereas he no longer does. Turning a fear of rejection into a drive to become a rebel turns any mainstream society repudiation into an affirmation of him being the rebel he wants to be. Of course, it is a defense mechanism and does not happen without some hesitancy.

He identified himself with the kid. Then he was accepted as a member of a bully group. "Because I had insecurities, you know, with my limping. I had insecurities. . . . And these bullies would protect you." He did not realize at the time that being a member of this group meant doing things he would not be proud of (e.g., bringing a girl's panties down). Together we explored whether feeling for the girl would make him another casualty of the bully group. When searching for protection, his group membership also made him their victim. His urge to become a rebel was a wish for freedom.

> Barbara Ehrenreich is a journalist and author. She wrote (about) the disappearance of women around age 45 from public view. They're gone. Only young beautiful women are publicized. If you look in the news, these women are stunning and beautiful. . . . A little bit fake-looking but, nevertheless, young and beautiful. But the average woman of 45–50 years is barely existent in the media. Chris Christie, the politician, the governor of New Jersey, is one of the big exceptions, but he is not very successful on a national level.

It is interesting that the subject of age was mentioned by Dr. Dillon, adding a man to his list of women disappearing from public spaces. Dr. Dillon is a professor. Four months previously he turned 52 years old and started to let his hair grow. Most of his life he was concerned about being fit. Now he was also afflicted by age. It might be that even when a person secures a position and relations, these are never firmly secured. A person could always be "eradicated" for their looks – for not complying with social values. This is remarkable in the sense that these social values appear totally reified, as if they were not set up by the members of our society and their practices. It could be that through fear of rejection people practice what they condemn. For Dr. Dillon "you cannot . . . I mean . . . throw away your culture, because your language sticks with you."

When I asked him what kind of things he does to fit in, Dr. Dillon said: "I like to fit in for my body so I take up cycling, but that throws me out of [the] loop of American culture because everybody has a car." This is a clear example of Dr. Dillon's capacity to face conflict and live within his principles, even at the cost of going against mainstream society. It shows the many circles, city-tribes, networks, and microcosmos available to any person, each group commending different virtues. At times, a person can find themself a member of different groups, all of which could hold contradictory values. For Dr. Dillon, a tribe "in the modern society, is basically a distinctive lifestyle which connects you to the others but also excludes others." Members of the "cycling tribe," as he called it, "might be very different, but riding a bicycle is . . . is what connects (you to) them." Dr. Dillon feels he has "an instant connection" whenever he encounters a fellow cycler just like him. "We say hello to each other. [Even if] I've never seen this person [before]." And as he said this, he suggested that nothing like that would ever happen between car drivers who had never seen each other before.

He admitted feeling guilty after driving a car that day. For the interview, he was forced to move into the microcosmos of car drivers, polluters of the air who challenge the principles he believes in and tries to live by. Becoming a bike rider transformed his life. It changed "my political attitudes. Joining the Green Party, being against the building of new interstates in Switzerland . . .

Uh! Against car traffic! Embracing public transportation. . . . All this, I mean, launched a lot in my life." His body "looks are actually fitting into it. I mean, uh . . . You're not overweight, you have good developed legs, um . . . You know. And you . . . I'm completely comfortable."

It is not enough to ride a bike. An occasional rider has an uneven pedal stroke that does not come from the hips, something that Dr. Dillon spots right away. He admits to only waving to riders such as himself. This is a narcissistic greeting that comes to confirm his well-being through the other, another just like him. As soon as he perceives a rider as belonging to "the inner circle of cycling," this rider comes to embody the values of the tribe for him. Dr. Dillon then is able to fuse himself with the ideal object. He feels the joy and pride of being a true member of the inner cycling tribe.

When asked about the other bicycle riders, Dr. Dillon admitted, "You're putting your fingers right in this wound." Those riders fail to support his image of integrity and well-being the way true riders provide. "I don't feel connected to them. . . . You know, that's the world. And I don't want to be connected to them. I don't want to talk to homeless people because I have these fears. . . . They will ask for money, they will ask me, you know, the typical thing. And I thought 'No.'" He envisions these distinct bicycle riders as being like the homeless. He associates them with individuals who have been eradicated from society. In his vision, they are a broken phallic symbol. They raise his castration anxiety. There is a sense of magic animism by which having contact with a homeless person would transform him into one of them. Contact is life creating, as when a mother holds a child. Later in life, there are things that can be touched and other things, like the penis, that are prohibited.

In general, the homeless are not integrated into society nor protected from the elements. Being integrated and protected are qualities Dr. Dillon praises. Indeed, being homeless would be an extreme example of what happens when someone is forgotten. In this case, ejected from society. It is possible to think, in the case of Dr. Dillon, that it has to do with his early feeling of abandonment from his biological father. Following his mentor, Dr. Dillon found a home in a foreign country.

As soon as he noticed his "close mindedness," he criticized himself. In an effort to be more open, he suggested he might say hello to those who have all the proper gear and don't look homeless. He might hail, hoping this person is on the way to becoming a member of the cycle tribe. "It's this kind of moralistic 'I'm better than you' attitude too. I mean there's some arrogance in it, you know. You know, you literally look down on car drivers," on those who do not belong.

Being a rider is a signifier that organizes his worldview. Dr. Dillon holds true cyclists at the top. Those who do not cycle from the hip but are "on the way to becoming true cyclers" are people who he might eventually be able to connect to. He despises homeless riders, and car drivers are at the bottom of his hierarchical social group. Being a rider is at the core of Dr. Dillon's sense of self. His worldview and political values are drawn from there. On a bike, he does not limp; he belongs. He is a peer, an equal to others. It is also a connection with a biological father that he only met later in life.

Only once was he mocked for his limping. He is perplexed by the fact that he has lived most of his life tormented about a belly he never thought he actually had and even feels innocent of (with doubts). Yet his very real imperfection, his limp, was never the object of mockery, something he was expecting to happen. He explained he was born with a clubfoot.

> So, my feet are not equal. I need special shoes. And you should expect that people will criticize you for that. But they didn't do that. Also, I was limping as a kid. I had a limp but that was. . . . I . . . I don't recall until in puberty when a youth gang, out in the city, uh . . . One of the guys was provoking a fight and he was aping my walk and exaggerating the limping and . . . But it's the only time somebody criticized me for that. Strangely enough, most people are supportive of that, which is a real physical problem I had.

When people show support, he is surprised. It becomes "a real physical problem" for him. As if he were more comfortable with condemnation than with praise. Early in his life, he failed to defend himself against the kid who teased him. "This episode, which stuck for the rest of my life with me, I bet it is completely gone from this man's consciousness. I don't think he would even remember it."

Notes

1 Results of the World Mental Health Surveys in 21 countries (Alonso et al., 2018) show a 12-month prevalence of DSM-IV anxiety disorder equal to 19.0% for the United States and 8.9% for Argentina. Furthermore, the World Health Organization (2018) identified depression as the leading mental illness worldwide.
2 The marriage rate is in decline in the United States and divorce is increasing. Divorce has tripled in those age 65 and older (Geiger & Livingston, 2019). New research established by Cigna (2108) shows that in America, 46% of individuals between 18 and 22 years of age feel the loneliest and express having no daily worthy interpersonal activities, such as having an extended conversation with someone.

8 Shame, body image, maternal function, and judgment

This book explores the results of a research study. I added clinical vignettes and personal experiences as we ventured into the topic starting from where we come from, as to what happens when things get complicated after feeling someone has judged us. The significance of early experiences and maternal care was made clear. This importance was also explored as the symbolic function of the Virgin Mary when considering the foci of the judgments and their effects. The Puritans colonized North America, but their rites did not include Mary. In the Puritan universe, adult males were a powerful authority. Females, natives and others were sources of sin, corruption or weakness (Chaplin, 2001/2003). Isolation of natives onto reservations and stratification of society by color are among the few things that followed. I suggested the Virgin Mary is an imago that could regulate the sadistic superego, which Bollas (2015) called the fascist mind. In the same manner, the maternal function needs to be regulated as well to allow exogamy to take place.

When talking about the body, I am not referring to the body of flesh and blood; rather the body we see and feel, and therefore it is a dyadic construction. By taking the body as a first object, the ego becomes the central reference point of consciousness, and the experience of belonging to a body is our sense of self. Again, that experience does not happen in a vacuum; it is anaclitically constructed first in relation with the mother[1] and from then on within social relations as suggested in Cooley's (1902/1922) definition of the self.

The mythical history of our lives in no way suggests that adults partake as children do. I am suggesting that there is a basic organization built upon emotional experiences an individual has during infancy and rediscovers and reelaborates throughout their life exchanges. The developmental description emphasizes maternal care. Both parents have an important role in a child growing up healthy.

Mother is a caregiving role. It is also a representation the child (or even a mature human) has – in the best of cases – of being desired and cared for. Our family is our first cultural matrix. That matrix is actively expecting the baby from before their birth takes place. The dyad is the second womb a mother provides to her newborn. It is home to potentiality as it functions within a framework of affective logic. Affect is a plus, a quantum of energy, the qualitative aspect which adds meaning to every thought and action provided by maternal care. Affective logic is preverbal, fused and fusing. The logic of affect never disappears. Rational thinking takes over with dominant power over emotions to secure safety and proper satisfaction by following the script of the reality principle. With maturity, knowing is to "be aware of through observation, inquiry, or information" ("Know," 2011), whereas understanding is to "perceive the intended meaning" ("Understand," 2011). Understanding comes with a plus, a quantum that indicates that the works of the affective logic can have an effect on cognitive discernment.

Mother is the first cultural agent an infant is exposed to. She interprets the child's needs and wants based on her personal, cultural, and aesthetic likings. Early belonging is supported on the taste values she provides through her appropriate actions and the experience of those actions felt by the child. I called them taste values, with no reference to the Kantian concept.

Later, belonging will involve a kind of cultural capital that both supports and sustains the social significance of a person, value that organizes the social ranking of individuals by separating members from outsiders. Dr. Dillon's narrative is a rich example of how he organized his social relationships, a pecking order that distinguished those who were able to offer him a reflective image by which he felt proud and worthy from those who left him feeling questioned, faulty, disregarded, or at risk of being cast-off as homeless people are. His rejection of the homeless was an effort to eliminate the feeling aroused by them, of coming into them. Of becoming ejected out of society, which is a threat always in the horizon of our lives.

Mother is her infant's first body, first face, and original refuge against all odds. The affective logic of the maternal function offers a sense of cohesiveness and consistency. Mother is not always readily available. Thus, an object close to the child comes to provide the needed comfort. The talents of the transitional object are a strategy to reach those qualities of what the child experienced within the dyad that is not readily found. That experience is a first frustration and initial boundary. The transitional object is an original me/not-me possession (Winnicott, 1971) that comes to provide the qualities of something that is lost but recreated. The child has not achieved the symbolic level when they start using this object. There is an archaic and presymbolic identification to that object. In Lacanian terms, the transitional object can be understood as a *petite object a* (Kirshner, 2005).

A transitional object provides cohesiveness and soothing experiences within the dyad. That soothing and sense of cohesiveness are acquired again at the symbolic level through identifying with the image a child finds in the looking glass. Transitional object and identification are narcissistic strategies to regain homeostasis. In both, the child identifies themself where they are not. Of course, there is a paradigm difference between Winnicott's and Lacan's theories

Unfortunately, entering into contact with the restrictions of reality is a constant frustration and abrasion. Not only that, the child also suffers attacks of partial objects from within. Eventually – once the child needs to rescind the object mother – the mirror offers an image the child takes as theirs, feeling like one in themself. That image brings a homeostasis that is no longer as dependent on someone else's action. That image has a background that is rich in family values that are taken at heart. During adolescence, in which social family relations are secondary to those the adolescent can create for themself, the sense of belonging takes a turn. The experience of being within the dyadic relationship is never forgotten. It is sought upon a sense of belonging once felt. It is a cherished added value to the self.

Transitional objects are in between what is real and what is phantasy, internal and external reality. For Winnicott (1971), the transitional object is decathected and "relegated to limbo" (p. 5). I suggest transitional objects do not become diffused but transformed, as is the dyad, to meet new developmental needs after achieving the symbolic level. A toddler reacts with frantic uneasiness when their transitional object has been displaced. Similar reactions can be found in an adult who has lost a cell phone.

Internal and external reality, phantasy and reality, are not spread apart. There is continuity, as in a Mobius figure. Transitional objects continue to exist in those things that have the distinct quality of being *mine*. Some things better than others, but most of our belongings are meaningful to us. They provide comfort. They help us maintain the illusion of being less precarious and to keep a better disposition throughout the ups and downs of any given day.

Among the counterphobic efforts that safeguard us from experiencing our castration: How many times do we dress up for an important meeting or bring with us something we feel we "need"? Unfortunately, daily frustrations tend to wear off the "magical powers" of these items. People shop for things they've seen in magazines or movies, or of a passerby who impressed them. As with the transitional object, they do so to procure the virtues of that impression for "social and psychological well-being" (Frater & Hawley, 2018, p. 300). Many buy celebrity memorabilia as a way of acquiring the essence of highly credited people. The price goes up or down in relation to the closeness of the celebrity's physical contact[2] (Newman & Bloom, 2014). The item not only provides comfort to the owner but also imparts higher grounds in their social hierarchy.

Mrs. Byer made her eyes up every morning after winning a contest for the most beautiful eyes at five years of age. She attunes the effect her presence has on others with an eyeliner. She feels her stunning blue eyes are a protective shield against criticism and discrimination. When a person is branded or typified (by self or others), their place and role in society is also defined. *Zelig* showed how the self is a façade of countless conscious and unconscious negotiations between internal and external needs that follow real, symbolic, and imaginary realms.

Via fantasized omnipotence and magical thinking, the dyad, the breast, the universe is the infant's creation. The dyad is not left behind. It is transformed. It is the source of our sense of belonging. Not every belonging means connection. Only when rich in affective logic can one make actual a sense of connection. Being desirable is at the base of the infant's survival. Indeed, it is at the base of everyone regardless of their age.

The part of the body participants were concerned about was a reminder of their primary insufficiency, their body morcellé, their lack, their being a freak. Shame is a feeling that raises the awareness of the denied limitations imposed by the fragmentation of our bodies and because we are a product of language. Being freaks makes us vulnerable and at risk of exclusion. The body boundary is the focus of terror and anxiety generated by the awareness of our mortality (Bauman, 2000/2018).

During the mirror stage, the child identifies with an image regaining a sense of being whole as first experienced in infancy. Such omnipotence was supported by the appropriate actions of maternal care. Utilizing the mirror, as Lacan's use of the can when he went fishing, the toddler sees themself where they are not and takes that position as theirs, thus becoming both an imaginary *not me* recognized as me, as the previously described *object petit a* as a transitional object, as well as a symbolic I.

At the mirror stage, mother confirms that image is her baby's, and in doing so, she sends a message of belonging. The child gains individuality. Yet the child can see mother as so much more, better, taller, idealized. Rage captures the child as they forever hatch out from the dyadic relationship to find its replacement in the sense of belonging. Rage is aggression turned inward, which thenceforth appears as shame, as a signal of disenfranchise to initiate restorative safeguarding actions to secure the relation. In shame, alienation and shunting act out the fear of rejection, which is the concern of repeating the first experience of loss within the dyad.

The body part that is the object of judgment assumes the burden of people's messages. It becomes somehow strange and threatening to their sense of self. Shame requires an act of sacrifice, by which a rejected aspect of the body is segregated to favor a more readily accepted self-image. Sacrifice is a private cleansing that helps transfigure into something acceptable or withal, something attractive.

Avoidant behavior is also a sacrifice performed to preserve the purity of the object and for self-preservation. It is not an attempt to save the object itself, but for the relationship that remains as a promise. The relationship that is the source of satisfaction for those who believe the drive satisfies itself through the path towards the object as Lacan (1964/1981) suggested when differentiating the drive's goal from its aim. That path is the link of our belongingness. This maneuver is regressive. Preserving the cathexis, safeguarding self and object, the relationship continues at the imaginary level as it has been done so many times.

Studies show that people with low levels of belonging tend to present fewer interpersonal relationships and higher life dissatisfaction (Mellor, Stokes, Firth, Hayashi, & Cummins, 2008). On the contrary, those who consider themselves as belonging tend to believe they are accepted by their peers, show lower levels of loneliness and use fewer medical services (Baskin, Wampold, Quintana, & Enright, 2010).

A few weeks ago, Cigna, the insurance company, sent me an email calling my attention to their research on increasing loneliness among younger generations. In 2018, 46% of individuals between 18 and 22 years of age felt the loneliest and expressed having no daily meaningful interpersonal activities (e.g., an extended conversation with someone). "Generation Z (adults ages 18–22) and Millennials (adults ages 23–37) are lonelier and claim to be in worse health than their older generations. Students have higher loneliness scores than retirees" (Cigna, 2018, p. 2). Moody (2001) found that social media can offer opportunities for social interaction while nonetheless making people feel increasingly lonely. He found that high degrees of face-to-face interaction with friends were associated with lower levels of emotional loneliness.

Putnam (2007) pointed out a drift towards individuality and community disengagement. At the liquid society, the sense of belonging is being redefined (Bauman 2000/2018). This is particularly the case in generations growing up exposed to virtual reality and the Internet. There is an entropic loss of the sense of connection and redefinition of what space means. Virtual communication fades geographic boundaries. As Ms. Ralph painfully admitted, sex is replacing love. Social bonds tend to be transient, precarious opportunities for instant satisfaction. Individuals live constantly redefining their personal criteria, deciding the autonomic guidelines to use in the constant creation and recreation of their subjectivity. Life practices, links, relationships, and views all tend to be more episodic than in previous generations that enjoyed long term security (Bauman, 2000/2018).

There was an upsurge in the worldview of uncertainty, insecurity, and indifference, especially after 9/11 (Bauman, 2000/2018; Philipson, 2010). Mass shootings remind us we are living in an era of terror. As Baudrillard (1991) described this era, "like viruses, (terror) is everywhere" (p. 20). This worldview turns individuality into a selfish shell to find refuge. "Hostility, competition, exclusion, indifference, insecurity, envy, and hatred" are deep in the cultural dynamics of our schools (Frank, 2013, p. 177). It is also found at home. "Self-hate arises when an individual complies with severely critical, abusive, or neglecting attitudes of important Others, often a parent. Self-hate describes the feeling of being inherently wrong, bad, inadequate, and not deserving of acceptance, protection, love, and happiness" (Gazzillo et al., 2018). Ms. Clayton is still unable to see the beauty I find in her, and she finds herself undeserving of a good job, a pleasant time, a trusting friendship.

Freud (1896/1953) conceptualized that at times the persecutory world in the selfish shell of individuality is nothing but our own reflection haunting us. Judgments, as negative self-talk are rather common. As Mrs. Hughes said, "Sometimes we can be our worst enemies. Negative thoughts are very easy to come into your mind," whether those thoughts are about ourselves or about others. When we expect the worst from others, any sign can be used to interpret antipathy and desertion as Mr. Whyte used to do.

Enjoyable social exchanges are protective factors against depression and many mental health disorders. They can be highly rewarding, provide support and nurturance, as well as protection against loneliness. Absence of belonging is a predictor of depression (Fischer, Overholser, Ridely, Braden, & Rosoff, 2015). Belonging is associated with increased self-esteem and higher academic, work and social achievements (Perry & Lavins-Merillat, 2019; Strayhorn, 2019).

Maybe there was a reduction in community engagement in the neighborhoods when Putnam (2007) wrote his classic book. By now, we have redefined what community is and are pretty mindful of the new ways of e-relating. We all spend hours communicating through computers, tablets, and smartphones, connected with a virtual reality yet disregarding the three-dimensional environment we live in. We can deeply criticize Harlow's studies. However, their research did indicate that a wire can never replace the warm sensation of bodies in dignified communion, a connection in which fitting together also means the peaceful equilibrium of both internal and external worlds. Harlow's research adds to what we have learned with Spitz's (1945) hospitalism, by which infants used to die from deprivation of love following birth. Being is belonging. Touching is a way of awakening the body. It is essential to feeling an emotional connection, to feel someone cares about us. To heal, we need to start by bringing and partaking in healing practices at home,[3] the supermarket, the parking lot, at work, and on the streets. Having positive moments at yoga class is not enough. Be the first one to offer a smile without any expectations. Eventually, you will be surprised by someone getting back at you with a positive gesture.

This study explored the effects of body-related judgments, whether real or imagined. Participants feared rejection and not being fit to fit in. The magnitude of the message's effect in participants' lives is puzzling when the messenger is described as inconsequential, almost as if the judgment was a result of projective identification, producing effects along the length of participants' lives. "I think that's sitting somewhere in the background of my head even if I'm not consciously aware of it," said Dr. Dillon, who ever since has avoided taking off his shirt in public and rides his bicycle 24 miles a day knowing it will help him "keep trimmed," as if the care provided to the body part would allow the building of a protective layer that both favors and resents how people feel others might judge them.

Judgments can be internalized, as the participants of this study have done. Those judgments spike at the truth of our denied fragmentation. Participants felt there was something wrong with them. They kept on treating the targeted part of their body in a defensive way in an attempt at managing their sense of self and sense of being in the world. Mrs. Teak reported not wearing rings to avoid getting attention or wearing rings to drive attention away from her hands, managing in this way her sense of self and desirability. Dr. Dillon and others wished to belong but feared being bullied or, simply said, spurned.

The judgments they felt subjected to were also systematically relational. In many occasions the world and social relationships were organized or filtered by real or imagined messages related to the given body part. Mrs. Hoocker, Mrs. Alem, and various participants classified social relations based on the attributes and meaning of their body experiences. Dr. Dillon described how he became a bully during his teenage years because he feared being bullied as a result of his limp. He was "grateful" to be admitted into a group. He felt protected from the torments of his own group, as well as from any bully group. It also meant doing things he continues not to be proud of. These conflicted feelings convey a prototype for social relations in which a person accepts a role that goes against their values in order to later feel grateful to and protected by the same group they abhor.

Several participants admitted to being their own authors of the judgment, which could be a way of controlling the message and its effects. Mr. Horowitz was the first one to joke about his nose so that others could not say anything he had not already remarked on. In any case, it seems the judgmental message can impact the body with high level of aggression and resonate at various levels. One of these levels is the idea of not being fit to fit in. Our primitive social world derives from the dyadic relation with the mother. Mother is the first source of emotional and taste values. Shame and shunting is breaking apart from later representatives of that safe haven.

By not being fit to fit in, a part of the body is then alienated. The judgment dismembers that part of the body, which becomes a focal point, representing the identity trauma of the individual. The message also carries a metaphor of a person's role in society. A sacrifice is offered to the gods to secure the bond, for good fortune, or to grant pardon. Even those who "wanted to be a rebel" wished to be part of the "inner circle," to use Dr. Dillon's words. There is a fear of ostracization, of not being allowed to become a member, of being left dismembered.

For the participants of the research and the clinical illustrations examined, negative judgments are like eating an apple and falling out of Paradise. Participants gave much attention to the body part in question. In that process, the body part assumed a central point of gravity in their identity trauma. I proposed that as guilt requires a reparative action, shame requires an act of sacrifice. The somatic phenomenon is someone's attempt at ego integrity and restoration of ties with social reality. The care provided to the body part is the result of countless negotiations made by the ego and powered by the pleasure principle, building in this way a protective layer that both agrees with and takes exemption to how people feel others might judge them.

St. Louis, August 24, 2019

Notes

1 Once again, mother, not as a person but as a narcissistic experience that happens within the dyad.
2 The price was found to go up in relation to how close the celebrity person was to the item, so long as the famous character had a positive standing in society. See Newman and Bloom (2014) for further details into their research study.
3 One of the things that surprised me when moving to the United States was finding that in many houses, living rooms are two recliners facing a television.

Glossary

Abjection   It is what is purged. When likeminded people bond following an idealized omniscient power that creates a strong boundary, they leave out all what do not fit – all that is not suitable to their rhetoric. It is a disruption of the natural symbolic order. All those pieces left out, excluded, or repudiated are the abject, the superego's object of gratification.

Acting out   A way of remembering in which thought is replaced by action. Freud discovered this phenomenon in patients who could not share memories through verbalization, which led him to examine the concepts of transference, repetition, and resistance in the analytic situation (see Freud's *Remembering, Repeating and Working Through*, 1914/1953).

Allocentric   Allo, from the Greek "other" (Klein, 1967). Allo-centric refers to having one's attention centered on other people. On the contrary, autocentric refers to a person whose focal point is on oneself.

Anaclitic   Means to "lean up against" in Greek. For Freud, object choice could be narcissistic or anaclitic. This second one is a resort of which mother is the primary embodiment. He recognized the anaclitic object choices as "the woman who feeds" or "the man who protects, and the succession of substitutes who take their place" (Freud, 1914/1953, p. 2945).

Aphanisis   Means disappearance in Greek. For Lacan (1981), aphanisis does not mean the disappearance of desire, but the disappearance of the subject (S11, p. 208). "The aphanisis of the subject is the fading of the subject, the fundamental division of the subject institutes the dialectic of desire (Lacan, 1981, S11, p. 221). Far from the disappearance of desire being the object of fear, it is precisely what the neurotic aims at; the neurotic attempts to shield himself from his desire, to put it aside" (Evans, 1996 p. 12).

Cathect   In the economic model of the mind, cathexis is investing psychic energy or libido on an object, "whether this is the representation of a person, body part, or psychic element" (de Mijolla-Mellor, 2005, p. 259).

Corps morcellé   Expression used by Lacan in reference to the fragmented body or body in pieces.

E-relating   Disembodied interpersonal relationship that happens in virtual reality and is mediated by any type of smart technological device.

Fragmentation   Freud would refer to annihilation anxiety. Kohut (1968) proposed fragmentation as opposite of cohesion of the self. For Kohut, fragmentation is a regression to autoerotism that announces the unstable configuration between mind, body, and self, thus triggering disintegration anxiety. Fragmentation occurs when the ego-structure is vulnerable, and can be experienced as an emptiness, low self-esteem, depression, anxious discomfort or panic, and fear of death. Fragmentation can also manifest in narcissistic rage (Kohut, 1977).

Gestalt   The synthetic function of the ego as a whole that is greater than the sum of its parts. According to Lacan, the total form of the body by which the subject identifies with in a looking glass, anticipates the level of maturation a child has achieved. Thus, the gestalt is only a powerful exteriority. "It symbolizes the mental permanence of the I, at the same time as it prefigures its alienating destination" (Lacan, 1971/2009a, p. 43).

Imago   More than an image or a representation, it is an idealized creation made in early childhood of a cathected love object. As idealized and omnipotent, it assists in regaining wholeness, cohesiveness, and consistency. Isaacs (1948) explained "the distinction between imago and image as: a) 'imago' usually refers to an unconscious image b) 'imago' usually refers to a person or part of a person, the earliest objects, whilst 'image' may be of any object or situation, human or otherwise; and c) 'imago' includes all the somatic and emotional elements in the subject's relation to the imagined person, the bodily links in unconscious phantasy with the id, the phantasy of introjection which underlies the process of introjection; whereas in the 'image,' the somatic and much of the emotional elements are largely repressed" (de Mijolla-Mellor, 2005, pp. 800–801).

Jouissance   Lacan (2009a) called *jouissance* the pleasure in suffering and symptoms, while Freud named it as the primary gain in illness, although these two things are not necessarily the same. Jouissance is pleasure beyond the limits of pleasure principle and desire is a defense against the jouissance. In desire, there is always a search for something else. (Evans, 1996).

Lack   In Freudian theory, each stage involves a loss that makes us unwhole. The oral stage, loss of the breast: anal stage, giving up the feces as a present; phallic stage, castration. Castration is universal. Girls don't have a penis, and boys experience their penis as a part of their body that is out of their control. In addition, the arbitrariness of language also results in a lack. For Lacan, the lack was primarily a lack of being. Lacan used the concept of the "lack" in distinctive ways: lack of having, which is associated with the demand lack of object, with castration being the most important of three types; and lack of a signifier in the Other, from which springs the search for meaning (Akhtar, 2009; Evans, 1996). "No matter how many signifiers one adds to the signifying chain, the chain is always incomplete" (Evans, 1996, p. 99).

Méconnaissance   A misrecognition that implies the difficulty in ever knowing who we are. For Lacan, the ego was a narrative construction. Due to the arbitrariness of the sign, the ego is also a symptom, an ongoing everlasting work of repetition and creation.

Mirror function   In Lacan's (1981) key concept of mirror stage or mirror phase phenomena, the child is captured by the illusion of oneness found in the reflection of their figure in the mirror. The mirror reflection helps maintain the illusion of wholeness due to the interplay of identification and projection. Any disruption in the mirror relation shatters the integrity of the child, who ends up experiencing what Lacan labeled "le corps morcellé," or fragmentation anxiety.

Mother   Mothering is a role and a responsibility. For the child, mother is an experience and, as such, is a representation of the experiences of having a mother. This definition does not attempt to undermine the importance of the biological mother.

Narcissism   The term was first used by Paul Näcke, but Freud borrowed this concept from Havelock Ellis to describe a variety of phenomena of the individual's concern to themselves. Although first considered a perversion, Freud (1914/1953) described it as "the libidinal complement to the egoism of the instinct of self-preservation, a measure of which may justifiably be attributed to every living creature" (p. 2,932). "Especially in persons whose libidinal development has suffered disturbance, their own selves are taken as the model. They seek themselves as a love–object and their type of choice of love-object may be termed Narcissistic" (Ellis, 1927, p. 138). Cathecting the body in the interest of self-preservation results in the creation of the ego. The libido withdraws from previous objects in order to take the body as an object. Thus, the formation of the ego is considered secondary narcissism. As the perfect harmony experienced within the dyad, the primary narcissism and the anaclitic first love, anaclitic love precedes object love. Freud also gave the example of how when someone suffers from a toothache, the cathexis returns narcissistically to the ego. The libido has a history. Thus, secondary narcissism implies introjection and identification. In *On Narcissism*, Freud (date) described four phenomena associated with narcissism: (a) as sexual perversion, (b) as a stage of development, (c) as a libidinal cathexis of the ego, and (d) as an object–choice. Narcissism can also be associated with the formation of the ego-ideal; and as a phase between autoerotism and object love. Finally, Kohut (1968) defined narcissism as cathexis of self-representations and as an agency in charge of issues of relationship (de Mijolla-Mellor, 2005, pp. 1105–1107).

Oceanic   Oceanic feeling is an experience of limitless, an all-embracing bond with the universe. Freud (1930/1953) borrowed the term *oceanic* from Romain Rolland; "It consists of peculiar feeling, which he himself is never without . . . a sensation of 'eternity', a feeling as of something limitless, unbounded – as it were, *oceanic*" (p. 64)

References

Abraham, K., & Lewin, B. D. (1966). *On character and libido development: Six essays*. New York, NY: Basic Books.

Akhtar, S. (2009). *Comprehensive dictionary of psychoanalysis*. London, UK: Karmac.

Allen, W. (Director). (1983). *Zelig* [Motion picture]. United States: Orion Pictures.

Allison, H. E. (2001). *Kant's theory of taste: A reading of the critique of aesthetic judgment*. Cambridge, UK: Cambridge University Press.

Alonso, J., Liu, Z., Evans-Lacko, S., Thornicroft, G., Evans-Lacko, S., Sadikova, E. . . . World Health Organization World Mental Health Survey Collaborators. (2018). Treatment gap for anxiety disorders is global: Results of the World Mental Health Surveys in 21 countries. *Depression and Anxiety, 35*(3), 195–208. https://doi.org/10.1002/da.22711.

Alperovitz, S. (2013). Nonverbal communication in analytic work. *Journal of American Psychoanalytic Association, 61*(2), 363–377.

Anzieu, D. (2007). *El yo-piel*. Madrid, Spain: Biblioteca Nueva.

Anzieu-Premmereur, C. (2015). The skin-ego: Dyadic sensuality, trauma in infancy, and adult narcissistic issues. *Psychoanalytic Review, 102*(5), 659–681.

Aragno, A. (2011). Silent cries, dancing tears: The metapsychology of art revisited/revised. *Journal of American Psychoanalytic Association, 59*(2), 239–288.

Armstrong, K. (2014). *The battle for God: Fundamentalism in Judaism, Christianity and Islam*. New York, NY: Harper Collins Publishers. (Original work published in 2000)

Aulagnier, P. (2015). Birth of a body, origin of a history. *International Journal of Psychoanalysis, 96*(5), 1371–1401.

Bacon, F. (2014). *Essays: Or counsels, civil and moral*. Auckland, NZ: The Floating Press. (Original work published in 1626)

Bartel, E. C. (2006). Too many blackamoors: Deportation, discrimination, and Elizabeth I. *Studies in English Literature, 46*, 305–322. https://doi.org/10.1353/sel.2006.0012.

Baskin, T., Wampold, B., Quintana, S., & Enright, R. (2010). Belongingness as a protective factor against loneliness and potential depression in a multicultural middle school. *The Counseling Psychologist, 38*(5), 626–651.

Baudrillard, J. (1991). *La transparencia del mal: Ensayo sobre los fenómenos extremos*. Barcelona, España: Anagrama.

Bauman, Z. (2018). *Liquid modernity*. Cambridge, UK: Polity Press. (Original work published in 2000)

Bavelier, D., Green, C. S., & Dye, M. W. G. (2010). Children, wired: For better and for worse. *Neuron, 67*(5), 692.

Bessell, A., & Moss, T. P. (2007). Evaluating the effectiveness of psychosocial interventions for individuals with visible differences: A systematic review of the empirical literature. *Body Image, 4*(3), 227–238. https://doi.org/10.1016/j.bodyim.2007.04.005.

Bethell, T. (1998). *The noblest triumph: Property and prosperity through the ages.* Houndmills, UK: MacMillan Press.

Bick, E., & Harris, M. (2011). *The Tavistock model: Papers on child development and psychoanalytic training.* London, UK: Harris Meltzer Trust by Karnac. (Original work published 1968)

Bisagni, F. (2009). The sound-hand. *Journal of Child Psychotherapy, 35*(3), 229–249.

Biven, B. M. (1980). The concept of a developmental network: Developmental pathways. *International Review of Psychoanalysis, 7,* 113–116.

Bollas, C. (2015). *Being a character: Psychoanalysis and self experience.* London, UK: Routledge.

Borges, J. L. (1976). Heraclito. In *Obras Completas.* Buenos Aires, Argentina: Emecé.

Bourdieu, P. (1984). *Distinction: A social critique of the judgement of taste.* Cambridge, MA: Harvard University Press.

Bowlby, J. (1958). The nature of the child's tie to his mother. *International Journal of Psycho-Analysis, 39,* 350–373.

Boyce, J. A., Kuijer, R. G., & Gleaves, D. H. (2013). Positive fantasies or negative contrasts: The effect of media body ideals on restrained eaters' mood, weight satisfaction, and food intake. *Body Image, 10*(4), 535–543.

Bradford, W., & Morison, S. E. (2016). *Of Plymouth plantation, 1620–1647.* (Original work published 1651)

Brigham, C. S. (Ed.). (2014). *British Royal proclamations relating to America 1603–1783.* Project Gutenberg. Retrieved from www.gutenberg.org/ebooks/46167. (Original work published 1911)

Campion, N. (2017). *The new age in the modern West: Counterculture, utopia and prophecy from the late eighteenth century to the present day.* London, UK: Bloomsbury Academic.

Cash, T. F., & Pruzinsky, T. (2002). *Body image: A handbook of theory, research, and clinical practice.* New York, NY: Guilford Press.

Chaplin, J. E. (2003). *Subject matter: Technology, the body, and science on the Anglo-American frontier, 1500–1676.* Cambridge, MA: Harvard University Press. (Original work published in 2001)

Chen, B., Van, D. R. M., Tan, C. S., Muller-Riemenschneider, F., Van, D. R. M., Chua, H. L., Wong, P. G., . . . Muller-Riemenschneider, F. (2019). Screen viewing behavior and sleep duration among children aged 2 and below. *BioMed Central Public Health, 19*–59.

Cherokee Nation v. Georgia, 30 U.S. 5 Pet. 1. (1831). Retrieved from https://supreme.justia.com/cases/federal/us/30/1.

Chiozza, L. (1999). Body, affect, and language. *Neuropsychoanalysis, 1*(1), 111–123.

Christenson, G. A. (2013). Liberty of the exercise of religion in the Peace of Westphalia. *Transnational Law & Contemporary Problems, 21*(3), 721–761.

Cigna. (2018). *Cigna 2018 U.S. loneliness index.* Retrieved from www.cigna.com/assets/docs/newsroom/loneliness-survey-2018-fact-sheet.pdf.

Clark, K. (2015). *Civilisation.* London, UK: John Murray. (Original work published 1969)

Connecticut. (1821). *The general statues of Connecticut with the constitution of the United States and the constitution of the state of Connecticut.* Hartford, CT: Huntington Jr. Press.

Cooley, C. H. (1922). *Human nature and the social order.* New York, NY: C. Scribner's Sons. (Original work published 1902)

Danielsson, I. M. B. (1999). Engendering performance in the late iron age. *Current Swedish Archaeology, 7,* 7–20. Retrieved from www.arkeologiskasamfundet.se/csa.

Darwin, C. (2018). *On the origin of species.* Minneapolis, MN: Lerner Publishing Group.

de Mijolla-Mellor, A. (2005). *International dictionary of psychoanalysis.* Detroit, MI: Thomson Gale.

Divozzo, R. J. (2019). *Mary for Protestants: A Catholic's reflection on the meaning of Mary the mother of God.* Eugene, OR: Resource Publications.

Donegan, K. (2002). As dying, yet behold we live: Catastrophe and Interiority in Bradford's of Plymouth plantation. *Early American Literature, 37*(1) 9–38.

Dreisbach, D. L. (2017). *Reading the Bible with the founding fathers.* New York, NY: Oxford University Press.

Driver, C. (2013). The 'holy mother' and the shadow: Revisiting Jung's work on the quaternity. *Journal of Analytical Psychology, 58*(3), 347–365.

Dunkelman, M. J. (2017). Next-door strangers: The crisis of urban anonymity. *Hedgehog Review, 19*(2), 44–57.

Durkheim, E. (2001). *The elementary forms of the religious life.* London, UK: Oxford University Press.

Dutch East Indian Company. (2019). *Encyclopedia compacta Britannica.* Retrieved from www.britannica.com/topic/Dutch-East-Indian-Company.

Ellis, H. (1927). The conception of narcissism. *Psychoanalytic Review, 14*(2), 129–153.

Erikson, E. H. (1980). On the generational cycle: An address. *International Journal of Psychoanalysis, 61,* 213–223.

Evans, D. (1996). *An introductory dictionary of Lacanian Psychoanalysis.* London, UK: Routledge.

Ex Parte Crow Dog. 109 U.S. 556. (1883). Retrieved from https://supreme.justia.com/cases/federal/us/109/556.

Feingold, A., & Mazzella, R. (1998). Gender differences in body image are increasing. *Psychological Science, 9*(3), 190–195.

Fischer, L. B., Overholser, J. C., Ridely, J., Braden, A., & Rosoff, C. (2015). From the outside looking in: Sense of belonging, depression, and suicide risk. *Psychiatry, 78*(1), 29–41.

Fisher, S., & Cleveland, S. E. (1968). *Body image and personality.* New York, NY: Dover Publications. (Original work published 1958)

Fisher, S. (1986). *Development and structure of the body image* (vols. 1, 2). Hillsdale, NJ: Lawrence Erlbaum Associates.

Foreman, G. (1989). *Indian removal: The emigration of the five civilized tribes of Indians.* Norman, OK: University of Oklahoma Press. (Original work published 1932)

Frank, D. B. (2013). A principal reflects on shame and school bullying. *Psychoanalytic Inquiry, 33*(2), 174–180.

Frater, J., & Hawley, J. M. (2018). A hand-crafted slow revolution: Co-designing a new genre in the luxury world. *Fashion, Style, & Popular Culture, 5*(3), 299–311.

Freud, A. (2018). *Normality and pathology in childhood: Assessments of development.* London, UK: Taylor and Francis. (Original work published 1965)

Freud, S. (1953). *The standard edition of the complete psychological works of Sigmund Freud* (J. Strachey, Ed.). London, UK: Hogarth Press and the Institute of Psychoanalysis.

Freud, S. (1981). *Sobre las teorías sexuales infantiles. Obras completas: Tomo 2 (1905–1917)* (L. Lopez Ballesteros, Trans.). Madrid, Spain: Biblioteca Nueva. (Original work published 1908)

Freud, S., & Jung, C. G. (1994). *The correspondence between Sigmund Freud and C.G. Jung 1906–1914.* (W. McGuire, Ed.; R. Manheim & R. F. C. Hull, Trans.). Princeton, NJ: Princeton University Press. (Original work published 1974). Retrieved from https://archive.org/stream/FreudJungLetters/The-Freud-Jung-letters-The-Correspondence-between-Sigmund-Freud-and-C-G-Jung_djvu.txt.

Gazzillo, F., Gorman, B., De Luca, E., Faccini, F., Bush, M., Silberschatz, G., & Dazzi, N. (2018). Preliminary data about the validation of a self-report for the assessment of interpersonal guilt: The Interpersonal Guilt Rating Scales-15s (IGRS-15s). *Psychodynamic Psychiatry*, *46*(1), 23–48.

Geiger, A. W., & Livingston, G. (2019, February 13). Eight facts about love and marriage in America. *FactTank*. Retrieved from www.pewresearch.org/fact-tank/2019/02/13/8-facts-about-love-and-marriage.

George-Tvrtkovic, R. (2017). Meryem Ana Evi, Marian devotion and the making of Nostra aetate III. *The Catholic Historical Review*, *103*(4), 755–781.

Goffman, E. (1963). *Stigma: Notes on the management of spoiled identity*. London, UK: Penguin Books.

Gogol, N. (2014). *The nose*. Brooklyn, NY: Melville House. (Original work published in 1836)

Gonzalez Taboas, C. (2017). *La Cita Fallida 1. El Continente Mestizo. Una mirada con Lacan*. Buenos Aires, Argentina: Grama.

Gregg, S. (2007). Legal revolution: St. Thomas More, Christopher St. German, and the schism of King Henry VIII. *Ave Maria Law Review*, *5*(1), 173–205.

Grimes, R. L. (2000). *Deeply into the bone: Re-inventing rites of passage*. Berkeley, CA: University of California Press.

Grogan, S. (1999). *Body image: Understanding body dissatisfaction in men, women and children*. London, UK: Routledge.

Haake, C. B. (2017). Civilization or savagery in the West? The west in Native American letters written during the removal era. *Amerikastudien*, *62*(1), 51–66.

Haarmann, H. (1998). The kinship of the Virgin Mary. *ReVision*, *20*, 3–17.

Hartmann, H. (1956). Notes on the reality principle. *Psychoanalytic Study of the Child*, *11*, 31–53.

Head, H., & Holmes, G. (1912). *Sensory disturbances from cerebral lesions*. London, UK: J. Bale, Sons & Danielsson.

Hobbes, T. (2013). *Leviathan, or the matter, form, & power of a common-wealth ecclesiastical and civil*. Literature Online Prose. Cambridge, UK: Proquest. (Original work published 1651)

Hofstede, G., Hofstede, G. J., & Minkov, M. (2010). *Cultures and organizations: Software of the mind* (Rev. 3rd ed.). New York: McGraw-Hill.

Horn, J. (2008). Why Jamestown matters: If the colony had collapsed the English might not have been established as the major colonial power in North America. *American Heritage*, *58*(3), 52–53.

Hume, W. T. (1892). *The laws and ordinances of the City of Portland, Oregon: Comprising the rules and order of business of the common council, rules and regulations governing the police and paid fire departments, charter of the city and all ordinances 1763–1970*. Portland, OR: Schwab.

Hutchinson, M. G. (1982). Transforming body image. *Women & Therapy*, *1*(3), 59–68.

Hyvärinen, L., Walthes, R., Jacob, N., Chaplin, K. N., & Leonhardt, M. (2014). Current understanding of what infants see. *Current Ophthalmology Reports*, *2*(4), 142–149.

Inderbitzin, L. B., & Levy, S. T. (2000). Regression and Psychoanalytic Technique. *Psychoanalytic Quarterly*, *69*(2): 195–223.

Isaacs, S. (1948). The nature and function of phantasy. *International Journal of Psychoanalysis*, *29*, 73–97.

Jackson, L. A. (1987). Gender, gender role, and body image. *Sex Roles*, *19*(7), 429–443.

Jacob, P., & Jeannerod, M. (2003). *Ways of seeing: The scope and limits of visual cognition*. Oxford, UK: Oxford University Press.

Jaimes, M. A. (1982). Towards a new image of American Indian women. *Journal of American Indian Education, 22*(1), 18–32.

James, B. B. (1904). *The history of North America: 5.* Philadelphia, PA: Barrie & Son.

Kant, I. (1790/2012). *Critique of judgement.* Mineola, NY: Dover Publications.

Karni, A., & Altman, L. K. (2019, February 14). At 243 pounds, Trump tips the scale into obesity. *New York Times.* Retrieved from www.nytimes.com/2019/02/14/us/politics/trump-obese.html.

Kent, G., & Keahone, S. (2001). Social anxiety and disfigurement: The moderating effects of fear of negative evaluation and past experience. *British Journal of Clinical Psychology, 40*(1), 23–34. https://doi.org/10.1348/014466501163454.

Kent, G., & Thompson, A. (2002). The development & maintenance of shame in disfigurement: Implications for treatment. In P. Gilbert & J. Miles (Eds.), *Body shame* (pp. 103–116). Hove, UK: Brunner-Routledge.

Kestenberg, J. S., Marcus, H., Robbins, E., Berlowe, J., & Buelte, A. (1971). Development of the young child as expressed through bodily movement. *Journal of the American Psychoanalytic Association, 19*, 746–764. https://doi.org/10.1177/000306517101900408.

Kirshner, L. A. (2005). Rethinking desire. *Journal of American Psychoanalytic Association, 53*, 83–102.

Klein, E. (1967). *A comprehensive etymological dictionary of the English language, dealing with the origin of words and their sense development thus illustrating the history of civilization and culture: Vol. 1: A-K.* London, UK: Elsevier.

Klein, M. (1990). *Obras completas.* Barcelona, Spain: Paidós Ibérica.

"Know." (2011). In *Concise Oxford English dictionary: Luxury edition* (A. Stevenson & M. Waite, Eds.). Oxford, UK: Oxford University Press.

Kohut, H. (1968). The psychoanalytic treatment of narcissistic personality disorders: Outline of a systematic approach. *Psychoanalytic Study of the Child, 23*, 86–113.

Kohut, H. (1977). *The restoration of the self.* New York, NY: International Universities Press.

Kristeva, J. (1982). *Powers of horror: An essay on abjection* (L. S. Roudiez, Trans.). New York, NY: Columbia University Press.

Kristeva, J. (1985). De la identificación: Freud, Baudelaire, Stendhal. In *El Trabajo de la Metáfora.* Barcelona, Spain: Gedisa.

Lacan, J. (1958). *Formations of the unconscious: Book V.* New York, NY: Norton.

Lacan, J. (1977). *La familia.* Rosario, Argentina: Homo Sapiens.

Lacan, J. (1978). *Seminar XXVI: Topology and Time: 1978–1979.* New York, NY: SUNY Press.

Lacan, J. (1980). *Seminario de Jacques Lacan: Libro XV: El acto psicoanalítico, 1967–1968.* Barcelona, Spain: Paidós.

Lacan, J. (1981). *The seminar of Jacques Lacan. The four fundamental concepts of psychoanalysis: Book XI.* New York, NY: Norton.

Lacan, J. (2006). *El seminario de Jacques Lacan: Libro I: los escritos técnicos de Freud: 1953–1954.* Barcelona, Spain: Paidós.

Lacan, J. (2007). *The seminar of Jacques Lacan: The other side of psychoanalysis: Book XVII.* London, UK: Norton. (Original work published in 1969)

Lacan, J. (2009a). *Escritos 1.* Buenos Aires, Argentina: Siglo XXI. (Original work published 1971)

Lacan, J. (2009b). *Escritos 2.* Buenos. Aires. Argentina: Siglo XXI. (Original work published 1975)

LaFantasie, G. W. (1988). *Review of the correspondence of Roger Williams* (Vol. 1). Hanover, NH: University Press of New England.

Laplanche, J., & Pontalis, J.-B. (2018). *The language of psychoanalysis*. London, UK: Taylor and Francis.

Lechte, J. (2003). *Key contemporary concepts: From abjection to Zeno's paradox*. London, UK: Sage Publications.

Lemma, A. (2010). *Under the skin: A psychoanalytic study of body modification*. London, UK: Routledge.

Lévi-Strauss, C. (1988). *Tristes Trópicos*. Buenos Aires, Argentina: Ediciones Paidós Ibérica. (Original work published 1955)

Liu, L., Yuan, C., Ding, H., Xu, Y., & Long, M. (2017). Visual deprivation selectively reshapes the intrinsic functional architecture of the anterior insula subregions. *Scientific Reports*, 7, 1. https://doi.org/10.1038/srep45675.

Lombard, A. S. (2003). *Making manhood: Growing up male in colonial New England*. Cambridge, MA: Harvard University Press.

Madley, B. (2017). *An American genocide: The United States and the California Indian catastrophe, 1846–1873*. New Haven, CT: Yale University Press.

Mariscotti, G. A. M. (1978). *Pachamama Santa Tierra: Contribución al estudio de la religión autóctona en los Andes centro-meridionales*. Berlin, West Germany: Gebr. Mann Verlag.

Marshal, H. E. (2011). *This country of ours* [Kindle DX version]. Retrieved from Amazon. com. (Original work published 1917)

Martinez Cerezo, A. (2014). La expulsión de los moriscos (1605–1618), según el Licenciado Francisco Cascales. *Revista Murgeteana, Real Academia Alfonoxo X el Sabio, 131*(LXV), 155–186.

Marx, K. (2014). *Economic & philosophic manuscripts of 1844*. Stilwell, KS: Neeland Media. (Original work published in 1932)

Masson, J. M. (Ed.). (1985). *The complete letters of Sigmund Freud to Wilhelm Fliess, 1887–1904*. Cambridge, MA: Harvard University Press.

McAdams, D. P. (2001). The psychology of life stories. *Review of General Psychology*, 5(2), 100–122. https://doi.org/10.1037/1089–2680.5.2.100.

McDaniel, X. C. (2019). The nation's unsettled account. *Smithsonian*, 50(5), 12–20.

McNeil, D. (1998). *The Face*. London, UK: Little, Brown & Company.

Mellier, D. (2014). The psychic envelopes in psychoanalytic theories of infancy. *Frontiers in Psychology*, 5, 734. https://doi.org/10.3389/fpsyg.2014.00734.

Mellor, D., Stokes, M., Firth, L., Hayashi, Y., & Cummins, R. (2008). Need for belonging, relationship satisfaction, loneliness, and life satisfaction. *Personality and Individual Differences*, 45, 3, 213–218.

Merleau-Ponty, M. (1958). *Phenomenology of perception* (C. Smith, Trans.). New York, NY: Routledge.

Money-Kyrle, R. (1978). *The collected papers of Roger Money-Kyrle*. Perthshire, Scotland: Clunie Press.

Moody, E. J. (2001). Internet use and its relationship to loneliness. *Cyberpsychology and Behavior*, 4, 393–402.

Nacht, S. (1952). The mutual influences in the development of ego and id – Discussants. *The Psychoanalytic Study of the Child*, 7, 54–59. https://doi.org/10.1080/00797308.1952. 11823152.

Nasio, J. D. (2008). *Mi cuerpo y sus imágenes*. Buenos Aires, Argentina: Paidós.

Newman, G. E., & Bloom, P. (2014). Physical contact influences how much people pay at celebrity auctions. *Proceedings of the National Academy of Sciences of the United States of America*, 111(10), 3705–3708.

Nice, G. (2014, October 15). *Human rights: Philosophy and history*. Retrieved from www. gresham.ac.uk/lectures-and-events/human-rights-philosophy-and-history.

Ogden, T. H. (2011). Reading Susan Isaacs: Toward a radically revised theory of thinking. *International Journal of Psychoanalysis, 92*(4), 925–942.

Paillard, J. (1999). Body schema and body image – A double dissociation in deafferented patients. In G. N. Gantchev, S. Mori, & J. Massion (Eds.), *Motor control: Today and tomorrow.* Sofia, Bulgaria: Academic Publishing House.

Paine, L. P. (2000). *Ships of discovery and exploration.* Boston, MA: Houghton Mifflin Co.

Pankow, G., & Goldstein, V. (1974). *El hombre y su psicosis.* Buenos Aires, Argentina: Amorrortu.

Perloff, R. M. (2014). Social media effects on young women's body image concerns: Theoretical perspectives and an agenda for research. *Sex Roles, 71,* 363–377.

Perry, J. C., & Lavins-Merillat, B. D. (2019). Self-esteem and school belongingness: A cross-lagged panel study among urban youth. *Professional School Counseling, 22*(1).

Philipson, I. (2010). Pathologizing twinship: An exploration of Robert Stolorow's traumatocentrism. *International Journal of Psychoanalytic Self Psychology, 5*(1), 19–33. https://doi. org/10.1080/15551020903384377.

Piaget, J. (1979a). *El mecanismo del desarrollo mental* (J. Delval, Ed.). Madrid, Spain: Editora Nacional.

Piaget, J. (1979b). *Seis estudios de psicología.* Barcelona, Spain: Seix Barral.

Piaget, J. (2013). *Child's conception of the world.* Taylor & Francis.

Pitron, V., Alsmith, A., & de Vignemont. (2018). How do the body schema and the body image interact? *Consciousness and Cognition, 65,* 352–358. https://doi.org/10.1016/j. concog.2018.08.007.

Porter, J. R., Beuf, A. H., Lerner, A., & Nordlund, J. (1986). Psychosocial effect of vitiligo: A comparison of vitiligo patients with "normal" control subjects, with psoriasis patients, and with patients with other pigmentary disorders. *Journal of the American Academy of Dermatology, 15*(2), 220–224.

Portman, T. A., & Herring, R. D. (2001). Debunking the Pocahontas paradox: The need for a humanistic perspective. *The Journal of Humanistic Counseling, Education and Development, 40,* 185–199. https://doi.org/10.1002/j.2164-490X.2001.tb00116.x.

Preester, H., & Knockaert, V. (2005). *Body image and body schema: Interdisciplinary perspectives on the body.* Amsterdam, Netherlands: J. Benjamins.

Putnam, R. D. (2007). *Bowling alone: The collapse and revival of American community.* New York, NY: Simon & Schuster.

Rapaport, D. (1996). *The collected papers of David Rapaport* (M. M. Gill, Ed.). Northvale, NJ: J. Aronson.

Real Academia Española (RAE). (2020). Sobre sexismo lingüístico, femeninos de profesión y masculino genérico. In *Informe de la Real Academia Española sobre el lenguaje inclusivo y cuestiones conexas.* Madrid, Spain: Espasa.

Reardon, M. J. (2012). *The bonds of manhood: Public life, homosociality, and hegemonic masculinity in Massachusetts, 1630–1787.* Dissertation. Retrieved from http://ir.uiowa.edu/etd/2969.

Riviere, J. (1936). On the genesis of psychical conflict in earliest infancy. *International Journal of Psycho-Analysis, 17,* 395–422. Retrieved from www.wiley.com/en-us/The+Internatio nal+Journal+of+Psychoanalysis-p-9780J.

Rizzuto, A. (2004). Roman Catholic background and psychoanalysis. *Psychoanalytic Psychology, 21*(3), 436–441.

The role played by protestant women in society from the XVIth to the XIXth centuries. (n.d.). Retrieved from www.museeprotestant.org/en/notice/the-role-played-by-protestant-women-in-society-from-the-xvith-to-the-xixth-centuries.

Rostand, E. (2009). *Cyrano De Bergerac: A play in five acts.* NetLibrary: Project Gutenberg. (Original work published in 1897)

Roudinesco, E. (2006). The mirror stage: An obliterated archive. In J.-M. Rabaté (Ed.), *The Cambridge companion to Lacan*. Cambridge, UK: Cambridge University Press.

Rubin, M. (2009). *Mother of god: A history of the virgin Mary*. New Haven, CT: Yale University Press.

Rumsey, N., Clarke, A., White, P., Wyn-Williams, M., & Garlick, W. (2004). Altered body image: Appearance-related concerns of people with visible disfigurement. *Journal of Advanced Nursing, 48*(5), 443–453. https://doi.org/10.1111/j.1365-2648.2004.03227.x.

Russell, S. (2002). Apples are the color of blood. *Critical Sociology, 28*, 65–76.

Saint-Exupéry, A. (2015). *El principito*. Salt Lake City, UT: Csorna Gutenberg Foundation.

Sami-Ali, M. (1984). *Lo visual y lo táctil*. Buenos Aires, Argentina: Amorrortu.

Sami-Ali, M. (1990). *El cuerpo, el espacio y el tiempo*. Buenos Aires, Argentina: Amorrortu.

Santoni-Rugiu, P., & Sykes, P. J. (2007). *A history of plastic surgery*. Berlin, Germany: Springer Berlin Heidelberg.

Santrac, A. S. (2017). The legacy of Martin Luther's Sola Fide. *In die Skriflig, 51*(11), 1–7.

Sartre, J.-P. (1984). *Being and nothingness: An essay on phenomenological ontology*. New York, NY: Washington Square Press. (Original work published in 1943)

Sartre, J.-P. (2001). *Jean-Paul Sartre: Basic writings* (S. Priest, Ed.). London, UK: Routledge.

Scambler, G. (2018). Heaping blame on shame: Weaponising stigma' for neoliberal times. *The Sociological Review, 66*(4), 766–782.

Schacht, R. (2017). *Alienation*. Hove, UK: Psychology Press.

Schachtel, E. G. (1961). On alienated concepts of identity. *The American Journal of Psychoanalysis, 21*(2), 120–131.

Schilder, P. F. (2014). *The image and appearance of the human body: Studies in the constructive energies of the psyche*. London, UK: Routledge. (Original work published in 1935)

Schneider, C. D. (1992). *Shame, exposure, and privacy*. New York, NY: W. Norton.

Schweik, S. M. (2009). *The ugly laws: Disability in public*. New York: New York University.

Silver, L. (2019). Smartphone ownership in advanced economies higher than in emerging. In *Smartphone ownership is growing rapidly around the world, but not always equally*. Pew Research Center. Retrieved from https://www.pewresearch.org/global/2019/02/05/smartphone-ownership-is-growing-rapidly-around-the-world-but-not-always-equally/.

Singer, T. (2010). The transcendent function and cultural complexes: A working hypothesis. *Journal of Analytical Psychology, 55*(2), 234–241.

Skeat, W. W. (1910). *An etymological dictionary of the English language*. Oxford, UK: Clarendon Press.

Skelton, R. (1995). Is the unconscious structured like a language? *International Forum of Psychoanalysis, 4*(3), 168–178. https://doi.org/10.1080/08037069508409542.

Solms, M. (2013). The conscious id. *Neuro-Psychoanalysis, 15*(1), 5–19.

Spitz, R. A. (1945). Hospitalism: An inquiry into the genesis of psychiatric conditions in early childhood. *Psychoanalytic Study of the Child, 1*, 53–74.

Spotnitz, H. (1961). The narcissistic defense in schizophrenia *Psychoanalytic Review, 48*(4), 24–42.

Stannard, D. E. (1994). *American holocaust: Columbus and the conquest of the New World*. Oxford, UK: Oxford University Press.

Stannard, D. E. (2006). *The Puritan way of death: A study in religion, culture, and social change*. New York, NY: Oxford University Press. (Original work published 1977)

Strayhorn, T. L. (2019). *College students' sense of belonging: A key to educational success for all students*. New York, NY: Routledge.

Sullivan, H. S. (1953). *The interpersonal theory of psychiatry*. New York, NY: Norton.

Symington, N. (1990). Religion and psychoanalysis. *Free Associations, 1*(19), 105–116.

Trull, T. J., Jahng, S., Tomko, R. L., Wood, P. K., & Sher, K. J. (2010). Revised NESARC personality disorder diagnoses: Gender, prevalence, and comorbidity with substance dependence disorders. *Journal of Personality Disorders, 24*(4), 412–426.

"Understand." (2011). In *Concise Oxford English dictionary: Luxury edition* (A. Stevenson & M. Waite, Eds.). Oxford, UK: Oxford University Press.

Ungar, V. (2012). Psicosomática Piel Clase 8: La importancia de la piel en la estructuración temprana del psiquismo. In *Trastornos dermatológicos en la infancia*. Buenos Aires, Argentina: Ed. Paidós.

Vance, W. R. (1924). The quest for tenure in the United States. *The Yale Law Journal, 33*(3), 248–271.

Vuola, E. (2019). *The Virgin Mary across cultures: Devotion among Costa Rican Catholic and Finnish Orthodox women*. Oxon, UK: Routledge.

Wieland, C. (2015). *The fascist state of mind and the manufacturing of masculinity: A psychoanalytic approach*. London, UK: Routledge.

Winnicott, D. W. (1965). *The maturational processes and the facilitating environment* (International Psychoanalytic Library, Vol. 64). London, UK: The Hogarth Press & the Institute of Psychoanalysis.

Winnicott, D. W. (1971). *Playing and reality*. London, UK: Tavistock Publications.

Winnicott, D. W. (1986). *Holding and interpretation* (International Psychoanalytic Library, 115:1–194). London, UK: The Hogarth Press and the Institute of Psycho-Analysis.

Wolfley, J. (2016). Reclaiming a presence in ancestral lands: The return of native peoples to the national parks. *Natural Resources Journal, 56*(1), 55–80.

World Health Organization. (2018). *Depression*. Retrieved from www.who.int/news-room/fact-sheets/detail/depression.

World Health Organization. (2019). Recommendations at a glance. In *To grow up healthy, children need to sit less and play more*. Retrieved from https://www.who.int/news-room/detail/24-04-2019-to-grow-up-healthy-children-need-to-sit-less-and-play-more.

Wurmser, L. (1997). *The mask of shame*. Northvale, NJ: J. Aronson.

Index

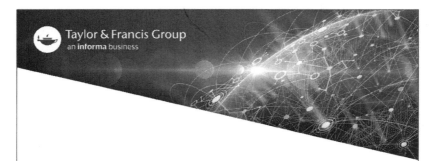
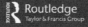